Primary Health Care
in Urban Communities

NATIONAL LEAGUE FOR NURSING SERIES

Home Health Outcomes and Resource Utilization Integrating Today's Critical Priorities   *Adams*

Curriculum Building in Nursing: A Process, Third Edition   *Bevis*

Community Activism and Health Care   *Burton*

Keepers of the Central Fire: Issues in Ecology of Indigenous People   *Colomeda*

Early Black American Leaders in Nursing: Architects for Integration and Equality   *Davis*

Learning Styles and the Nursing Profession   *Dunn*

Case Studies in Cultural Diversity   *Ferguson*

Educating the 21st Century Nurse: Challenges and Opportunities *Ferguson*

Culture, Curriculum and Community   *Fitzsimmons*

Nurse Educators 1997 Findings from the RN and LPN Faculty Census   *Louden*

Profiles of the Newly Licensed Nurse, Third Edition   *Louden*

Patterns of Rogerian Knowing   *Madrid*

Annual Review of Women's Health, Volume III   *McElmurry and Parker*

Primary Health Care in Urban Communities   *McElmurry, Tyska, and Parker*

Guide for the Development and Management of Nursing Libraries and Information Resources   *Moore*

The Emergence of Family into the 21st Century   *Munhall*

Hope: An International Human Becoming Perspective   *Parse*

Writing-to-Learn: Curricular Strategies for Nursing and Other Disciplines   *Poirrier*

Evidence-Based Teaching   *Stevens*

Teaching in the Community: Preparing for the 21st Century   *Tagliarini*

Jo Ann Ashley: Selected Readings   *Wolf*

Asian Voices: Asian and Asian American Health Educators Speak Out   *Zhan*

Primary Health Care in Urban Communities

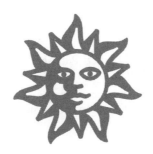

Beverly J. McElmurry, EdD, FAAN
Cynthia Tyska, MA
Randy Spreen Parker, RN, C, PhD
with the assistance of
Todd Hissong, BS

JONES AND BARTLETT PUBLISHERS
Sudbury, Massachusetts
BOSTON   TORONTO   LONDON   SINGAPORE

World Headquarters
Jones and Bartlett Publishers
40 Tall Pine Drive
Sudbury, MA 01776
978-443-5000
info@jbpub.com
www.jbpub.com

Jones and Bartlett Publishers Canada
2100 Bloor Street West
Suite 6-272
Toronto, ON M6S 5A5
CANADA

Jones and Bartlett Publishers International
Barb House, Barb Mews
London W6 7PA
UK

PRODUCTION CREDITS
ACQUISITIONS EDITOR   Greg Vis
PRODUCTION EDITOR   Linda S. DeBruyn
MANUFACTURING BUYER   Kristen Guevara
DESIGN   Argosy
EDITORIAL PRODUCTION SERVICE   Argosy
TYPESETTING   Argosy
COVER DESIGN   Ben Lenz
PRINTING AND BINDING   Braun-Brumfield

Library of Congress Cataloging-in-Publication Data
Primary health care in urban communities / [edited by] Beverly J.
  McElmurry, Cynthia Tyska, and Randy Spreen Parker.
    p. cm.
    Includes bibliographical references and index.
    ISBN 0-7637-1010-5
    1. Primary health care—Illinois—Chicago. 2. Community health
  services—Illinois—Chicago. 3. Community organizations—Illinois—
  Chicago. I. McElmurry, Beverly J. (Beverly Jane) II. Tyska,
  Cynthia. III. Parker, Randy Spreen.
    [DNLM: 1. Primary Health Care—Chicago. 2. Urban Health Services—
  Chicago. 3. Community Health Services—organization &
  administration—Chicago 4. Community Networks—organization &
  administration. W 84.6 I619 1999]
  RA427.9.I58   1999
  362.1'09773'11—dc21
  DNLM/DLC
  for Library of Congress   98-52867
                                                             CIP

Cover photographs by William Harder

Printed in the United States of America
02 01 00 99   10 9 8 7 6 5 4 3 2 1

This book is dedicated to Ms. Gwendolyn Pinager
of the University of Illinois at Chicago's Office
for International Studies—
"the glue that keeps it all together."
As we maintain and facilitate numerous projects,
Gwen keeps the staff sane and organized
while also serving as a strong, caring,
and resilient role model for students
and community women alike.
We are in her debt.

Foreword

BY DR. HELEN K. GRACE

Reviewing this book has given me the opportunity to revisit a number of issues related to working with people to improve their well-being. In the late 1960s I first met one of the women who later became a health advocate. Mary Bell has contributed to this book, and continues to work on behalf of the Southside Chicago community in which she lives. As a community mental health faculty member of the University of Illinois at Chicaco College of Nursing, I worked with community members and students who taught me some of the most important lessons that have shaped both my professional and personal life. Sitting in discussions in church basements, eating in the restaurants in the community, and working with people in high-rise public health complexes brought me to a world I had only known from a distance, and one that I feared. Perhaps the most important lesson that was learned as we worked in the community was not to be afraid, and to meet people on their home ground—in their homes, churches, and in the highways and byways of their lives. People who became community advocates, like Mary Bell, were my most valuable teachers, and the lessons learned were much more cogent than hours spent in classrooms and in theoretical discussions, although both are needed.

When I later became dean of the College of Nursing at the University of Illinois at Chicago, several faculty members who were developing a research and practice field related to women's health began to raise their concerns over the distance between the university and the inner-city communities that surrounded it. As they become involved with community groups, such as the Mexican- and African-American communities around the university, they recognized the need for "translators—not only of language but intermediaries between the 'professionals' and the 'community.'" While the means of financially supporting this important work were extremely limited, the faculty persevered and the results represent the outgrowth of years of development and work on the part of committed faculty members, staff from an array of agencies, and most important, people from the community who have become true advocates on behalf of their communities.

As I reviewed this manuscript, I was struck by our need for a language that describes working together. Our language is replete with connotations of hierarchy, status, power, and control while limited in terminology adequate to describe partners working together for a common end. "Professionals," "patients or clients," "advocates," and "empowering" or "developing" people (implying that someone has power to give or that people can be developed), "providers" and "receivers," "majority" and "minority." The contributing authors of this book have made a giant step forward in documenting and describing the lessons learned from the work with community advocates in a variety of settings. In a world in which coinage of politically correct language has often become a code, I encourage those who read this book and share a concern for establishing a new ground for working together to look closely at the language we use, and to search for clarity and a language that more adequately conveys working together on a common ground. Each party brings to the table different expertise, life experiences, and skills. Teamwork involves bringing the diversity represented in individual team members together into a whole that works effectively toward common goals.

This book is an important account of the training of community health advocates and the evaluation of these programs has wide application in an array of settings, both nationally and internationally. As concerns continue to rise over the cost of health care, and in particular health care for the poor and disenfranchised, ways of bridging the gap between communities and healthcare "systems" become increasingly important. When the poor seek medical care, it is usually a desperate measure when all else has failed. Going into the stark environment, being treated as less than a human being, and rushed out the door with a prescription or advice that is not easily understood is hardly conducive to developing health practices that might avert medical crises. Community health advocates working in the community, actively educating people about sound health practices, and working to bridge the gap between people and those who work in the healthcare field can be effective in making a difference. But the gains to be made are long range, rather than immediate. And therein lies a major dilemma. In the current frenzy to "cut costs," the methods used are those that can only increase cost in the long run—unless people simply die in their tracks. Homicide and suicide are the most efficient cost-cutting measures known. But in a so-called civil society these are hardly acceptable as explicit means of cost control. Costs of chronic illnesses, of drug and alcohol addiction, of inappropriate use of resources, both physical and human in our healthcare systems—these are the long-range concerns that can only be addressed by bringing together communities and healthcare givers into collaborative work. Key to building this form of collaboration is engaging community members to be bridgers and communicators across the boundaries of the disparate worlds in which we live and work.

Contributors

Rachel Abramson, RN, MS, IBCLC, The Chicago Health Connection

Ellen Barton, RN, MS, Circle Family Care, Chicago, IL

Karen A. Buck, MS, University of Illinois at Chicago College of Nursing

Aaron G. Buseh, MPH, RN, Evaluation Consultant, The Chicago Health Corps

Carol Christiansen, PhD, University of Illinois at Chicago College of Nursing

Peg Dublin, RN, BSN, Program Manager, The Chicago Health Corps

Patricia Fox, PhD, University of Illinois at Chicago College of Nursing

Benn Greenspan, MPH, President and CEO, Mount Sinai Hospital Medical Center, President and CEO, Sinai Health System, Chicago, IL

Ada Mary Gugenheim, BA, Program Officer, Senior Staff Associate, The Chicago Community Trust

Todd Hissong, BS, Communications Specialist, The Chicago Health Corps

Agatha Lowe, PhD, RN, Director of Women and Children's Health Programs, City of Chicago, Department of Public Health

Sybil Massey, Director of Grants Management, The Chicago Department of Public Health (CDHP)

Beverly J. McElmurry, EdD, FAAN, Professor, Public Health Nursing, and Associate Dean, Office for International Studies, Univeristy of Illinois at Chicago College of Nursing. Dr. McElmurry was Principal Investigator for the Primary Health Care in Urban Communities project.

Jeretha McKinley, BA, IBCLC, The Chicago Health Connection

Maureen Meehan, MA, Literacy Specialist, Literacy for Health project

Gloria T. Meert, MA, Program Director of Health and Programming, W. K. Kellogg Foundation, Battle Creek, MI

Susan J. Misner, MSN, RN, Health Educator, University of Illinois at Chicago College of Nursing

B. Joan Newcomb, PhD, RN, Program Coordinator, University of Illinois at Chicago College of Nursing

Kathleen F. Norr, PhD, Project Evaluator, Primary Health Care in Urban Communities project, University of Illinois at Chicago College of Nursing

Chang Gi Park, PhD, University of Illinois at Chicago College of Nursing

Randy Spreen Parker, RN, C, PhD, University of Illinois at Chicago College of Nursing

Susan M. Poslusney, RN, PhD, Assistant Professor, Department of Nursing, DePaul Univeristy, Chicago, IL

Francisco Ramos, Founding Member, Centro San Bonifacio, Chicago, IL

Lori Ramos, MA, MPH, Executive Director, Centro San Bonifacio, Chicago, IL

Jacqueline Reed, MA, Director, Westside Health Authority, Chicago, IL

Julio Rodriguez, Director of Community Resources and Development, The Governor's Task Force on Human Services Reform, Chicago, IL

Rosario Sanchez, Community Health Promoter and Program Coordinator, Centro San Bonifacio, Chicago, IL

Linda Diamond Shapiro, MSW, MBA, Director, Program Planning and Policy, Sinai Family Health Centers, Chicago, IL

Cassia Soares, RN, MPH, University of Sao Paulo, Sao Paolo, Brazil

Joanna Su, Mutual Aid Associations' Women's Health Education Project, Chicago, IL

Susan M. Swider, PhD, RN, Associate Professor, School of Nursing, St. Xavier University, Chicago, IL

Cynthia Tyska, MA, Doctoral Candidate, University of Illinois at Chicago College of Education

Virginia Warren, RN, MS, University of Illinois at Chicago College of Nursing

Mayumi Anne Willgerodt, MS, University of Illinois at Chicago College of Nursing

Contents

Chapter 1

Introduction to Primary Health Care in Urban Communities

BEVERLY J. MCELMURRY
with the assistance of
TODD HISSONG

This book really started over a decade ago when a graduate nursing student challenged a faculty member identified with women's health to "walk the talk." (In actuality, the challenge was worded somewhat more bluntly!) The discussion between the student and the faculty member revolved around the plight of inner-city women when they tried to access health services for themselves or their family. Initially, the focus of this discourse was on ways to reform the system of healthcare to allow low-income women to have a voice. When a fearless program officer from a local foundation (Ada Mary Gugenheim of the Chicago Community Trust) developed the initiative called Chicago Health System Reform, the response to the student's challenge was "Why not?" And therein lies a tale we will never be able to adequately describe in words. However, this book is written with the same attitude: Why not try to give voice to what we have learned? As the wise counselor she is, Gloria Meert (our program officer for the W. K. Kellogg Dissemination Grant that made this book possible) opined that putting examples into print offers the reader ideas to try in their own setting.

To that end, this book begins with one of the initial projects funded by the Chicago Community Trust to prepare nurse/health advocate teams for work in two low-income Chicago communities, one African American and one Hispanic American. For us, the main focus in that project was to develop a strategy that prepared community women to work with health professionals. We found that most of our work took us down the path of grassroots or community-based development primarily for two reasons: First and foremost was our commitment to women's health, particularly that of inner-city women and their families. A second reason was a realistic assessment of nursing's position within a health sciences center. We questioned our ability to garner support from other health professions within that center to agree to a reorientation to community-based health initiatives. In that respect, and as a primarily female occupation, nurses within a high-tech health center could identify with the lack of empowerment in the health system faced by community women. Our work in primary health care (PHC) and preparing community health workers (CHWs) actually began before there was readily available literature on this topic. Since then, others' experiences with CHWs in the United States have been more frequently reported in the literature, and various groups have defined what is meant by CHWs (CDC, 1994).

Internationally, the CHW's role has been an integral part of the PHC approach to achieving Health for All. The CHA role in the inner city corresponds to the CHW role in underdeveloped countries. Over time, we evolved a description of CHAs that works for us:

Community Health Advocates

Community Health Advocates (CHAs) assist communities to improve health via individual and community action directed at: improving living conditions; becoming aware of and using healthcare resources;

and making healthy life choices. The CHAs work with residents of their communities to gain control over their health and lives.

Experience indicates that this process works best when a CHA is a resident of the community in which s/he works. As a community resident, the CHA is aware of community concerns, sensitive to community issues, and comfortable in the surroundings. Generally, an Advocate is noted for leadership qualities and has a strong desire to effect positive change within the community. Although an Advocate may not have formal education beyond high school, s/he is articulate, intelligent, and skilled in interpersonal communication. Individuals who are selected for this role by members of their communities have close ties to their neighbors and are effective in mobilizing community residents to address shared health concerns.

Through the training process, CHA trainees develop and strengthen the knowledge and skills necessary to work with their neighbors. The Advocate training program covers a variety of health-related topics including: assessing and maintaining community health, maternal-child health, alcohol and substance abuse, and domestic and community violence. Included in many of the sessions are opportunities for personal sharing. Throughout the training series, a variety of role-playing scenarios are conducted, many of which are drawn from actual experiences of CHAs. Through the sharing of their unique concerns, each CHA trainee is a contributing part of a self-taught community. A successful CHA is a unique combination of personal strengths, community characteristics, and training.

CHAs work in teams with a public/community health nurse. While the work varies, throughout the process of training and subsequent employment, an effort is made to tie the work to the "essential elements" of PHC as defined by the World Health Organization (WHO). These elements include, but are not limited to: health education; maternal-child health, including family planning; immunizations; proper nutrition; basic sanitation and housing; prevention and control of locally endemic diseases; treatment of common illnesses and injuries; and provision of essential medications. Among other things, CHAs have worked on finding emergency food and housing, organizing people to improve housing or street safety, teaching nutrition and first aid, and speaking for the community at public forums on health-related issues. Many CHAs are actively involved in community coalitions. The role/function of the CHA within the community is that of a lay health teacher, information and health provider, and community organizer. Continuing education and counseling is provided on a routine basis to help CHAs address community-specific health issues.

Overall, the CHA role is one of a bridge between the community and the formal health system, an informed source of consumer health information, and a person skilled in supporting and empowering community residents to increase self-reliance in, and community control over, their health (OIS, 1997).

In 1996, Elsa Koch, a health policy analyst, offered a status report on community health worker programs in the United States (Koch,1996). Much of her assessment mirrors our experience in implementing change (Swider & McElmurry, 1990; McElmurry et al., 1990; McElmurry, Swider & Norr, 1991; Bless, Murphy & Vinson, 1995; McElmurry et al., 1995; McElmurry et al., 1997). Based on our locus in an academic institution that prides itself on research achievements, we have always asked how our work contributes to scholarship. That is, as members of the nursing profession and in our position as a WHO designated Collaborating Centre for the Advancement of Primary Health Care, how does our work promote the involvement of communities in the decisions that evoke improvement in essential healthcare? In reflecting on this question, we were assisted by WHO documents that articulate the university role in PHC as one of technical assistance to improve the public's access to acceptable, appropriate, and affordable healthcare (Bless et al., 1995). As opposed to being peripatetic consultants, we take the position that using various demonstrations and interventions is critical to helping people in the university and community understand the essence of PHC. Within the university, we garner criticism from those who think provision or management of services is inappropriate in institutions where the primary mission is education and research. However, we continue to believe that such practice settings are the source of research questions and important vehicles for reality-based education. The community poses a much more basic question, and one with which we eternally struggle: "What will happen when you leave?" To that we have many responses based on the context of their situation. If we have a sense that the community can sustain some activities, we identify that strength to them. The best of all possible worlds is one in which community residents take the reins of the initiatives while we facilitate the process until it is sustainable over time. However, when we fall short of that goal, we sometimes have to content ourselves with "better something than nothing."

LINKING HEALTH PARTNERS

After we had some experience in preparing and launching nurse/advocate teams we turned to the question of enhancing collaborative decision making regarding health concerns. In Figure 1, we depict the interaction of professional, community, and health service environments.

Eventually, we described the work of health advocacy collaboration with health professionals and health systems reform within the PHC framework. And, over time, we learned how to use PHC as a philosophy, process, and/or system perspective in healthcare delivery and economic development. Given

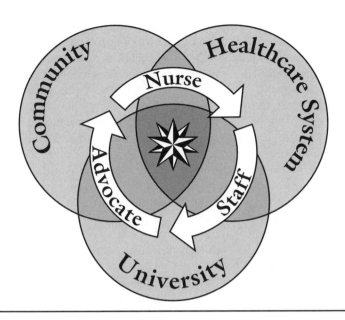

FIGURE 1.
Interaction of PHC Partners

that PHC is an evolving concept for all participants, an abbreviated definition describes our perspective.

Primary Health Care

Primary Health Care is a pattern of healthcare delivery in which the community residents and health professionals are partners in achieving the common goal of improved health. Primary health care (PHC) uses the strategies of community participation, transfer of appropriate technology, public education for health, decentralization, and coordination across geographic or social sectors (intersectoral coordination). These strategies are directed toward achieving the long-term goal of Health for All by the Year 2000 (HFA/2000). The Health for All movement was launched in 1977 with a resolution adopted by the Thirtieth World Health Assembly. The HFA strategies are characterized by the processes of self-learning, self-determination, self-care, and self-reliance on the part of the people.

The implementation of PHC emphasizes several concepts: (a) accessibility of health services to all of the population; (b) maximum individual and community involvement in the planning and operation of healthcare services; (c) emphasis on services that are preventive and promotive rather than curative; (d) the use of appropriate technology with local resources and government support; (e) the integration of health development with total overall social and economic development; (f) provision of culturally acceptable health activities; and, (g) a focus on the health concerns of highest priorities for the community residents and health system.

Primary care, as often used in the United States, defines a mode of health delivery which adopts a psychosocial, ecological model focused on the individual and the family. Primary care coordinates the care an individual requires over time and emphasizes disease prevention and health promotion and recognizes the care of problems and diseases in early stages. Thus, the four "C's" of primary health care are often said to be: (first) contact, continuous, comprehensive, coordinated care. Primary care can be seen as a subset of primary health care where primary care concentrates on the users of health services (the numerator population) and primary health care focuses on the community (denominator population).

Overall, PHC is an approach to health care which focuses on the promotion of health and the prevention of diseases, through comprehensive care which is collaboratively and cooperatively provided by community people and multiple disciplines. Primary health care is interactive: Community residents are empowered to be knowledgeable in health matters and to have an opportunity to participate in their health care management. Moreover, PHC addresses self-care practices for physical and mental aspects of community health as well as community social and environmental conditions. A basic goal is to ensure that PHC is available to everyone in the community (OIS, 1997).

We have endured some teasing from colleagues who maintain that when you adopt the tenets of PHC it may be time to resign. By that same token, we have learned survival tactics from others who have been less friendly to some of our ideas. Most of the time we have moved forward (and backward, and sideways) with the attitude that a moving target is harder to hit than a stationary object. The concept of resilience is something those committed to PHC understand emotionally and experientially. Consequently, we have seen many positive developments in the years that we have worked in community-based PHC. We have observed that emerging ideas often represent a confluence of forces and people in many areas. In this case, people are worried about the lack of basic universal healthcare for all people as well as the great disparities in healthcare and morbidity/mortality rates for different groups. Currently, we are optimistic that the environment in which we work has moved to an understanding that there is value in articulating a university's relationships to its communities (Stukel, 1993).

Trying to maintain funding for a community-based program of scholarship requires a great deal of work from tremendously talented groups of staff and support persons. To outsiders, a PHC program of work and funding does not always make sense. Some have accused us of "going where the money is," and there may be a grain of truth in such criticism. We accept the accusations without apologies because we have maintained our integrity by proposing PHC initiatives that made sense to us, were consistent with our philosophy of PHC, and kept a momentum alive. This financial challenge to maintaining grassroots, community-anchored innovations was corroborated in Sally Lundeen's description of the initiation and development of a Chicago community health center (Lundeen, 1986). Financing innovation or the equivalent of a community-based research and development health program remains a struggle, for some of the most exciting innovations in the community are "loosely" described as community-based health programs. Most of the grassroots or PHC community services piece together a response to health concerns that more established and long-term agencies have not embraced. A sample of the mix of research, education, and service activities that have engaged us are presented in Table I (Appendix A).

For this book we have included some projects that are closely identified with the University of Illinois at Chicago (UIC) as well as some that are not. However, the potential for ties and interactions between projects in a large urban area are both rewarding and frustrating. When people can come together for sharing and collaboration the outcome is exciting. Unfortunately, a more realistic view is the fact that the crises of the day take precedence over collaborative dialogue toward shared goals. This continues to be one of the greatest challenges for the future.

We hope our efforts to capture some of what we and our colleagues have done will prove helpful to others. The chapters were written within the context of community participation in PHC through partnerships among a variety of agencies and organizations. The following authors present a rich and varied pattern of health activity. In the next chapter, we present a panel discussion that addresses what it will take to maintain community-based projects in this day and age when funding mechanisms for health are rapidly changing. All of the panelists came to the topic with rich backgrounds in public and private organizations and work to advance healthcare innovation in response to human needs. They represent the diversity of views that are found in the current health scene.

In Chapter 3 Soares, Swider, and McElmurry describe how the health advocates were selected and trained, and explore the CHA's feelings about the experience. The education of community women as health advocates was a central theme of the Primary Health Care in Urban Communities (PHCUC) Project based in two Chicago communities; one whose population is primarily African American and the other Hispanic American. In each community, PHC was implemented through a CHA/public health nurse team approach. The authors also discuss the evaluation component of the program which used a Freiriean-based participatory approach consistent with our work and the tenets of PHC. Based on data acquired through a knowledge questionnaire, interviews, training session observations, and a focus group, evaluation results are presented and their implications discussed along with recommendations.

In Chapter 4 , Norr, McElmurry, and Misner have captured the voice of the CHA by presenting an analysis of recorded focus groups and discussions held with CHAs over several years. Our retrospective effort involved identifying themes that emerged in conversations and judging the "fit" between those themes and the PHC perspective we hold about the overall purpose of our work in community-based activities. The hope is that as the advocates describe their role in the community (with all of its satisfactions and frustrations), the reader finds the CHA's voice as compelling as we did. Over time, the CHAs generated a distinctive view of their "team" (the community, university, and the healthcare system) which proved to be especially enlightening. As we have always observed, the advocates found the experience to be life changing, a feeling that was shared by those of us who were lucky enough to work with these wonderful women.

A nurse/CHA team's work with Hispanic immigrant women is described by Buck and Fox in Chapter 5. Hispanics immigrating to the United States face many challenges to their health as a result of being in an unfamiliar country with a different language, culture, and sociopolitical system. Since 1991, a nurse/CHA team has worked to empower Hispanic immigrants in four Chicago areas to improve health and development. The authors undertook a qualitative exploratory study to describe a sample of Hispanic immigrant women involved in the program. The women participated in one-on-one interviews with the first author and described their interaction with the CHA. Their comments were assessed to determine if their descriptions reflected empowerment. The importance of relationships emerged as the overarching theme and as the means of empowerment for these women.

The evaluation of PHC projects presents many challenges. In Chapter 6 Norr and McElmurry discuss key issues in evaluation, and suggest strategies for resolving them using examples from the PHCUC project. To maximize the benefits of program evaluation, the varied stakeholders in PHC projects must be considered and involved in the evaluation process. While a participatory evaluation model is conceptually compatible with the goals of PHC, such a model requires strategies to capture the structure, function, processes, and integrity of a community-based PHC program.

Another perspective on the previous project, Door-to-Door (State Legalization Impact Assistance Grant or SLIAG) is presented in Chapter 7 by Park and Warren. The authors detail a healthcare outreach service to selected Latino immigrant communities in Chicago that focuses on the nurse/CHA team and how their interdependent roles provide an effective model for implementing PHC services. Door-to-Door identifies families and individuals with multiple complex needs and assists them in accessing community services. The authors describe a six-step process whereby the nurse/CHA case-management team provides assistance to overcome barriers, promote the community as a resource, and promote family self-reliance and informed self care. The project demonstrates that interacting with immigrant families to help them gain access to health and social services promotes greater health provider accountability to underserved Latino immigrant communities.

In Chapter 8 McElmurry, Meehan, and Buseh illustrate the concept of health literacy and the process of developing an adult learning program to improve the health outcomes of inner-city residents as well as their competencies in using and interpreting written health information. Health literacy is an extension of basic literacy in that it is a functional set of skills applied in everyday life through such tasks as making nutritional decisions, using medications, following and interpreting written medical advice, and completing health information forms. The curriculum was taught through a whole-language approach to literacy development and addressed three types of literacy: prose, quantitative, and documentary (using charts, tables, etc.). The curriculum built on the learner's experiences and skills and emphasized contextually meaningful written material. It was taught by a public health nurse and an experienced CHA from an inner-city community with support from university personnel. The teaching style emphasized participation of both learner and teacher in the learning process and encouraged class discussion and collaborative learning. The authors discuss how the concept of PHC guides the curriculum and presents strategies for implementing the curriculum in other community settings.

The Chicago Health Corps, a university-based AmeriCorps program, is described in Chapter 9 by Dublin. She pays particular attention to PHC training for community residents and health profession–bound students with an emphasis on the development of a community service ethic. The purpose of the Health Corps is to improve access to quality comprehensive PHC services by supporting collaborative, community-based service efforts. Health Corps participants assist their communities in reaching people who face barriers in accessing healthcare, and develop an awareness of the needs of their fellow community members. The project represents an alliance of Chicago area health and education organizations to annually enlist about forty Chicago area residents, 17 years and older, in a year-long program of community service. The author describes activities of the Health Corps and the transformations Members experience during their term of service.

In Chapter 10, Reed describes the Austin Community Wellness Initiative, an effort to rebuild communities through matching capacities. The Westside Health Authority is a community-based coalition in Chicago's Austin community that was formed to build and support community residents and organizations. The initiative grew out of efforts to address mistrust and fear of exploitation, work at ways to build bonds among neighbors, and rebuild community health and well-being through a focus on sharing, caring, and giving among neighbors. Using the community capacity building model, the Wellness Initiative both identified the capacities of community residents and developed programs and activities through which they could be shared. The Wellness Initiative in the Austin community was built on a vision of people loving, trusting, and sharing with each other and mobilizing community involvement through capacity building. The example of programs tried in the Austin neighborhood should be of interest to residents of any community.

Community-based healthcare centers and their practitioners can be instrumental in changing both the community as well as health professions education. In Chapter 11, Barton describes PHC in an urban teaching community health center. Here, health is viewed as an outgrowth of social, political, and economic conditions that influence individuals, families, groups, and communities. Healthcare delivery in underserved areas requires unique strategies to handle complex social and health problems, harness strengths within families, and create effective networks between programs and communities. The perspectives of public health, PHC, and capacity building are used to promote programs and activities that address serious health problems. A university affiliation enables the community health center to provide quality, reality-based educational experiences for health professions students, and research relevant and useful to both the center and community. The author demonstrates that teaching community health centers located in underserved communities prepare healthcare students with the skills necessary to work effectively with high-risk communities, and increase the access of community residents to healthcare.

In Chapter 12, Building Healthy Latino Communities, Ramos, Sanchez, and Ramos describe the efforts of Centro San Bonafacio, a community-based organization committed to implementing strategies that build healthy Latino communities in an urban setting. Consistent with PHC, the center's philosophy is grounded in the belief that members of the community must act as the main protagonists in the quest for health and well-being. Key strategies include women's education and empowerment, disease prevention, maternal and child health, traditional wisdom and medicine, and community organizing. From its inception, the center's focus has been on self-empowerment and leadership development which has resulted in a strong commitment to peer health promotion through the training of neighborhood residents as community health promoters. The authors describe in detail how a community coalition based on ethnicity and shared goals can effectively empower residents to realize personal and community development.

The work of the Chicago Health Connection (peer education for maternal/child health) is described by Abramson in Chapter 13. A central philosophical commitment of the project is women speaking for themselves. The author describes how Frierian principles of education and community guide the project's approach to community building. Strategies for health promotion involve not only training CHAs to support other women, but also training and working with various professional staff and institutions. Over time, project staff have learned that when community members speak for themselves, health, leadership, and economic development are profoundly affected in a positive way. Readers will gain an appreciation of the complexity of forming effective collaborative partnerships between health professionals and community members, specifically the challenge of giving voice to all stakeholders in community-based health promotion efforts.

Peer education for AIDS prevention in multiethnic non-English-speaking communities is described in Chapter 14 by Willgerodt, Christiansen, and Su. The Mutual Aid Association's Women's Health Project was established in 1994 as an effort to increase access and understanding of preventive PHC services among immigrant and refugee women. The authors describe the AIDS prevention project within the context of partners whose aim is to increase AIDS awareness and prevention through the peer education model. Planning, implementing, and evaluating PHC programs in non-English-speaking communities poses unique challenges for healthcare professionals. This chapter addresses these challenges and offers recommendations for future program planning.

In Chapter 15, PHC for Urban School Children, Newcomb illustrates how the concepts of PHC guide the development of comprehensive health programs in several Chicago elementary schools. Multidisciplinary teams of health professionals (nurse, pediatrician, dentist) collaborate with school personnel and school CHAs to tailor each school's program to the unique needs and interests of the school community. This is an especially appropriate approach in urban areas where there is economic, educational, and cultural diversity that mitigate against a "one size fits all" service design. The author elaborates on how the role of the school CHA is valuable in linking the healthcare providers with communities and in interpreting community values and concerns.

The PHC curriculum, grades K–8, is described in Chapter 16 by McElmurry, Newcomb, Lowe, and Misner. The purpose of this project was to develop, implement, and evaluate an age- and needs-appropriate PHC curriculum for school-aged children and their families through engaging community residents, school personnel, and students in the identification of health concerns. The authors describe a culturally sensitive health education curriculum that is useful in teaching health promotion and maintenance as well as self-management skills. The ten health-related themes are presented along with the major topics covered in each grade. The authors discuss the lessons learned over time and strategies for implementing a PHC curriculum in schools.

The healthcare system in Chicago (in fact, throughout the nation) has changed dramatically during recent years, a process that has seen many health providers experience ownership changes, often several times in a short period. Shapiro and Greenspan describe an example of one such change in Chapter 17, Healing Bodies and Building Lives: One Hospital's Model for Change. Many institutions have altered or abandoned their original mission, while others have lost the connection between hospitals and their communities, a connection that was critical in the formation of most health institutions in the United States. Sinai Health System implemented a model of town meetings to discuss ways the health system and community residents can address some of the most pressing health problems facing urban communities. The authors summarize the lessons gleaned from these town meetings, and this chapter furnishes a stimulus for other health systems across the nation to reflect on the strengths they provide to their communities and seek collaborate strategies to heal and build.

In Chapter 18, Poslusny describes the transformational leadership development emphasized in one PHC program. To promote PHC as a strategy to achieve "Health for All," the Leadership for PHC project enabled enhancement of the capacity for leadership in socioeconomically disadvantaged communities through collaborative partnerships between university personnel and community residents. As an action learning program for grassroots community leaders and community-based health professionals, this year-long program included a curriculum for transformational leadership development in PHC, a teaching/learning process designed to promote critical awareness, and support for community innovation and health policy development. Discussed in this chapter are program highlights and outcomes, obstacles encountered in developing such programs, key characteristics of transformational leaders, and implications for improvement in health status.

We conclude this book in Chapter 19 with McElmurry, Parker, and Tyska describing some of the lessons learned from PHC based on our experiences, conversations with participants, and work with the authors of the various chapters. Our efforts to highlight selected PHC projects has confirmed the importance of trying to anchor scholarship in the realities faced by urban residents. With every project, every new initiative, there has been yet another lesson to be learned, another insight to be gained. Yet there is also great vitality in the work reported by our colleagues. We hope you find this book useful and challenging.

REFERENCES

Bless, C., Murphy, D., & Vinson, N. (1995). Nurses' role in primary health care. *N&HC: Perspectives on Community, 16*:2, March/April 1995.

Community health advisors: Models, research and practice (Selected annotations, Vol I), and *Community health advisors: Programs in the United States* (Program descriptions, Vol II). (1994). Atlanta, GA: HHS, PHS, CDC.

Koch, E. (1996). *Promotoras and community health advisors: Program challenge in an age of change.* Washington, DC: Project on Sustainable Changes, Harrison Institute, Georgetown University Law Center.

Lundeen, Sally P. (1986). University of Illinois at Chicago Health Sciences Center. *Nursing reality survival: An organizational analysis of a nurse managed neighborhood health center.* Ann Arbor, MI. DAI, Vol. 47–083, p. 3295.

McElmurry, B., Swider, S., Bless, C., Murphy, D., Montgomery, A., Norr, K., Irvin, Y., Gantes, M., & Fisher, M. (1990). Community health advocacy: primary health care nurse-advocate teams in urban communities. *Perspectives in nursing,* 1989–1991. National League for Nursing, New York, NY, Publication #41-2281.

McElmurry, B., Swider, S., & Norr, K. (1991). A community-based primary health care program for integration of research practice and education. *Curriculum revolution: Community building and activism.* National League for Nursing Press, New York, NY, Publication #15-2398.

McElmurry, B., Tyska, C., Gugenheim, A. M., Misner, S., & Poslusny, S. (1995). Leadership for primary health care. *N&HC: Perspectives on Community, 16*:4, June 1995.

McElmurry, B., Wansley, R., Gugenheim, A. M., Gombe, S., & Dublin, P. (1997). The Chicago Health Corps: Strengthening communities through structured volunteer service. *Advanced Practice Nursing Quarterly*, *2*(4), 59–66, Aspen Publishers Inc.

Office for International Studies (1997). Definitions of "community health advocates" and "primary health care." Unpublished works. Available from the University of Illinois at Chicago College of Nursing, 845 S. Damen Ave. (M/C 802), Room 1158, Chicago, IL 60612.

Stukel, J. J. (1993). The University of Illinois at Chicago's new direction: Addressing urban needs. Chicago, IL: UIC Great Cities Program, pp. 1, 2, 10.

Swider, S. & McElmurry, B. (1990). A women's health perspective in primary health care: A nursing and community health worker demonstration project in urban America. *Family Community Health*, *13*(3), 1–17. Aspen Publishers Inc.

World Health Organization (1984). The role of universities in the strategies for health for all: A contribution to human development and social justice. Geneva, Switzerland: WHO (Resolution WHA 37.31, 20 pp.)

APPENDIX A

TABLE 1.
Selected Demonstrations of Primary Health Care—
UIC College of Nursing

Project Title	Funding Agency	Years	Project Description
Community Health Advocacy	The Chicago Community Trust	1987–1991	To demonstrate PHC approach to improving community health via the nurse/advocate team (application of nurse/advocate model).
Collaborative Decision Making	The W. K. Kellogg Foundation	1989–1992	To expand demonstration of PHC approach via education of health professionals and community residents to work together; facilitate university-community collaboration (education/ practice/ evaluation).
Social Policy Component	The Robert R. McCormick Charitable Trust	1989–1992	To enhance PHC efforts via adding staff with social policy expertise to work with nurse/ advocate teams and faculty (social policy Component).
UIC Nation of Tomorrow/ Partners in Health	The University of Illinois at Chicago	1989–1993	To establish the nurse/advocate team in four inner-city schools (multidisciplinary practice model).

TABLE 1. (CONTINUED)
Selected Demonstrations of Primary Health Care—
UIC College of Nursing

Project Title	Funding Agency	Years	Project Description
Child Passenger Safety Seat	Illinois Department of Transportation	1990–1992	To expand range of health issues addressed by a nurse/ advocate team, and to educate state agencies about health concerns of inner-city communities (essential PHC services).
REACH Futures	The Healthy Tomorrows partnerships between the USPHS Office of Maternal and Child Health, American Academy of Pediatrics, Harris Foundation, UIH	1990	To provide health promotion home visits by maternal-child health advocates (MCHAs) to women and infants in areas of high infant mortality (application of model for special focus on maternal-child health).
Peer Education for AIDS Prevention in Botswana	National Institute on Aging/U.S. Agency for International Development	1990–1993	To test and demonstrate a cultural adaptation of the peer education model for AIDS prevention in Botswana.
Healthy Sons, Healthy Families Conference	DHHS, Office of Minority Health	1990–1991	To encourage collaboration between health professionals and community residents around minority, male health issues (education about minority health issues).

TABLE 1. (CONTINUED)
Selected Demonstrations of Primary Health Care—
UIC College of Nursing

Project Title	Funding Agency	Years	Project Description
Leadership for Primary Health Care	The W. K. Kellogg Foundation	1990–1994	To design and implement a program for leadership development in PHC in partnership with community residents and health professionals.
PHC for Newly Legalized: Hispanic Health Coalition	DHHS, Office of Minority Health contract with the Chicago Department of Health, and Chicago Department of Health subcontract to UIC	1991–1996	To provide CHA/ nurse teams to underserved, hard-to-reach populations (access to essential PHC services) and to promote application of health advocacy concepts and PHC approach in coalition with health agencies in Hispanic communities (dissemination of PHC and development of case management approach).
Maternal-Child Health Advocacy Training	Mayor's Office of Employment and Training	1991	To train ten PHC advocates for work with nurse/advocate teams for the Chicago Department of Health (sustainability of model and training program).

TABLE 1. (CONTINUED)
Selected Demonstrations of Primary Health Care—
UIC College of Nursing

Project Title	Funding Agency	Years	Project Description
PHC for Urban School Children	Robert Wood Johnson Foundation	1992–1995	To improve school based-linked access to PHC care for children and their families, including expanding the multidisciplinary team and project evaluation (practice, education, and evaluation).
PHC in Urban Communities/ Immunization	Blue Cross/Blue Shield	1992–1994	To demonstrate that health advocates as members of immunization teams on mobile care vans increase immunization of children in public housing (multiple agency collaboration).
Health Literacy in the Inner City	National Institute for Literacy	1992–1993	To implement a concept of health literacy based in the nurse/advocate model which improves the health outcomes of inner-city residents and their competency in using and interpreting written health information (university/ community partnership).

TABLE 1. (CONTINUED)
Selected Demonstrations of Primary Health Care—
UIC College of Nursing

Project Title	Funding Agency	Years	Project Description
Language Services for Immigrants	Traveler's and Immigrant Aid	1992–1993	To improve client access to health care by documenting Cook County healthcare agencies provision and use of interpreter and translation services (public policy).
Health Literacy in the Inner City	Fry Foundation	1993–1994	Expand use of nurse/advocate model to implement a health literacy program for inner-city residents that enhances competence in writing and reading.
PHC Curricula, Grades K–8	Otho S. A. Sprague Memorial Institute	1993–1996	To increase the access of youth to health care and achieve the participation of community residents and school personnel in health education programs (education/practice).
Institutional Research Training Program in PHC	NIH, NINR	1994–1999	Support research training in PHC for predoctoral and postdoctoral trainees. Special emphasis on community-based research with special populations and models for the delivery of PHC services.

TABLE 1. (CONTINUED)
Selected Demonstrations of Primary Health Care—
UIC College of Nursing

Project Title	Funding Agency	Years	Project Description
Minority International Research Training	NIH, Fogarty International Center	1994–1999	To provide support for undergraduates, faculty, and graduate trainees from minority groups in the United States to conduct PHC research in an international setting.
Chicago Health Corps: an AmeriCorps Project	The Chicago Health Consortium subcontract to the UIC College of Nursing	1994–1999	To offer a year-long program of community service designed to improve access to quality comprehensive PHC and related services by supporting collaborative, community-based service efforts (alliance of Chicago area health and education organizations).
Healthy Cities Conference/ Great Cities Seed Funds	Montgomery Ward Foundation	N/A	To introduce the Healthy Cities concept in a one-day conference on the Healthy Cities movement in the United States for 100 Chicago participants (dissemination).

TABLE 1. (CONTINUED)
Selected Demonstrations of Primary Health Care—
UIC College of Nursing

Project Title	Funding Agency	Years	Project Description
PHC For Urban School Children	The W. K. Kellogg Foundation	1995/ 1998	To demonstrate a comprehensive PHC school-based/linked program for essential healthcare services in the community areas of two Chicago public schools (policy, practice, sustainability).
Dissemination of PHC	The W. K. Kellogg Foundation	1995/ 1997	To distribute information about recent experiences with primary health care projects developed by individuals and groups in Chicago (dissemination).
Planning the Evaluation of a PHC Curriculum Component: The Teacher/ Parent Participants	UIC Center for Urban Education, Research & Development	1995–96	To interview selected public school teachers regarding their readiness for use of the PHC K–8 curriculum (evaluation).
PHC High School Curriculum	Catholic Health Alliance of Metropolitan Chicago	1997–1999	To develop and present an age- and needs-appropriate PHC curriculum for female students in a private high school (education).

Chapter 2

Primary Health Care & Public Policy: A Panel Discussion

ADA MARY GUGENHEIM
SYBIL MASSEY
GLORIA T. MEERT
JULIO RODRIGUEZ
LINDA DIAMOND SHAPIRO

In October 1996 a panel of healthcare and policy experts were assembled at the University of Illinois at Chicago College of Nursing to discuss "Community-Based Projects in the New Era of Health Care Funding." The panel consisted of: Ada Mary Gugenheim from the Chicago Community Trust; Sibyl Massey from the Chicago Department of Public Health; Gloria Meert from the W. K. Kellogg Foundation; Julio Rodriguez from the Illinois Governor's Task Force on Health Care Reform; and Linda Diamond Shapiro from Sinai Family Health Centers. A brief bio and description of the participants and their organizations follows at the end of this chapter. Prior to the event, the Primary Health Care Dissemination staff formulated and submitted a set of questions to the panelists for their response. The diverse views these panelists brought to the table captured many of the issues that have made healthcare reform in the 1990s so challenging. What follows is an edited transcript of the discussion.

Question: Respond to the following quote: "With so much agreement about public/private partnerships, why is there so little progress? Why do we see these themes reflected in discreet local programming, both inside and outside the public and private sector, but not across large-scale public systems, and not as part of widespread comprehensive and collaborative systems? Why is the rhetoric so hard to make real?" (Walker, 1996)

Julio: Business practices focus providers on how they are held accountable rather than how the services they're delivering are actually meeting the needs of their communities. But providers and the government have to start to think to themselves, "Who is your customer? Do the consumers of your services really understand what it is you're attempting to do? Have we clearly set outcomes that everyone agrees are the outcomes that the state of Illinois wants to achieve in its human service systems?" I would say at this point we have not. We are still looking at categorical ways of just funding problems. We are not necessarily working with families in entireties. We divide families up based on the problems that we prescribe. We are not necessarily using our dollars in the most efficient and beneficial ways that our communities would prefer. Does the community really understand what it gets for its investment? Does it really understand how human service dollars, which is one-third of the state's budget (over $12 billion) really translate into meeting the needs of communities?

Sibyl: The Chicago Department of Public Health has been selected by the Department of Housing & Urban Development as one of the lead agencies responsible for

Empowerment Zones. We have the charge of meeting with community-based organizations and consumers to determine how the money is going to be used in communities. We try to sit at the table not only with private agencies, but with consumers to determine what directions we should go in. From a historical perspective, I think that we're being forced to change our thinking. In the 1960s, there was a lot of money poured into cities and states under model cities and Equal Employment Opportunity efforts to enhance programs in the community. In the '80s and early '90s there were federal cutbacks to these programs, and I think at present we have not kept up with those changes. Community characteristics have changed, consumers have changed the way that we deliver services. I think that people basically have to come back to the table and be educated about the way things are in the '90s.

Linda: What I thought this quote was about was a euphemism for MediPlan Plus, our state's mandatory Medicaid managed care program for Medicaid beneficiaries. This represents a massive transformation of a public program into a publicly supported private sector initiative. Considering the economics that have driven MediPlan Plus, I question whether there's any economic incentive that will work to indeed make this a neighborhood sensitive, responsive program. Some of the program's innovations look promising. One of the hallmarks of Medicaid managed care programming is that large, for-profit HMOs can diffuse Medicaid providers to places where they've never been before. The problem of provider participation in Medicaid changes dramatically when large systems place providers where they're needed. But will we have a comprehensive and collaborative neighborhood system as a result? I think some re-focusing will be necessary to accomplish this.

Gloria: I don't think anyone realizes the difficulties of forming partnerships and collaborations until they get involved with it. John McKnight says, "We know better than we do," and I think when we start talking about rhetoric, that's the part of knowing, and doing is the reality. Our public systems have been established to carry out categorical funding, thus fragmenting the delivery of services. We really need to look at how public/private partnerships can come together by asking "What's the common ground?" Communities know what their problems are and the solutions. How do we bring them to the table and find that common ground? Some questions that need to be considered in forming the partnerships are: What are the risks involved for the communities, the university, and the public organizations? When they come together in partnership each will bring something. The community will bring its own way of knowing, their wisdom, and what they can contribute to the partnership. The public systems bring their resources and their expertise. Both have something to gain but it's finding the balance of how to work together to make for more meaningful programs and services for families and communities where the challenge lies.

Mary: I think that there is a great deal of agreement about public/private partnerships in the way we operate health systems in this society. The fundamental way in which we deliver human services is essentially a public/private partnership. For instance the Medicare program, which we've now had for some thirty years, is a perfect example— there's a public revenue stream that pays for privately delivered services: some not-for-profit, some now proprietary, and some professional partnerships which is how most medical services physicians were organized originally when the program started. An example in Illinois would be the Ounce of Prevention program where one very knowledgeable philanthropist put up private sector money to do something differently twenty years ago. He then managed to influence large public revenue streams from the state to follow his ideas, and the program continues to flourish.

If we look at fundamental programs for meeting basic human needs, such as the services offered by the Salvation Army, somewhere between 50 and 60 percent of their budget comes from public sources, but the control and management of these programs is done by the private sector, by a lot of volunteer effort on the part of boards, which form the governing structure of these organizations, and by a professional staff that works in the not-for-profit organized agency.

When it comes down to the idea of widespread comprehensive and collaborative neighborhood systems, I claim it doesn't work at that level, because there is no mandate in this country to create it.

Question: How do you shift perspective more and more to community-based programs?

Sibyl: I think it would help to clarify what we mean when we talk about community-based programs. What is "public?" What is "private?" I work for the city and we have numerous health centers in communities. We're in the trenches, but people tell me that we're not community based, that we're governmental or private.

Mary: I think you've hit on a very key issue. We go on talking about it and using the same set of words without defining them. Until we re-define the terms and agree what we're talking about, we're not going to get any further in this debate. I take huge exception to the notion that "community" is a code word meaning the poor, or inner-city, or minority populations. People who live in an affluent suburb are a community. It's a community that has perhaps different problems.

Since most healthcare recipients in the private or public sector have such little control over their healthcare and benefits, let's get beyond the false divide and say, "the community" should be the whole pool of all of us and we should all be treated in the same pool. On the whole, other societies have managed to do it. Perhaps we could start defining one set of standards and argue locally about how the services were organized.

Julio: When we say the term "community," we also often think about it in terms of geographical boundaries that are set up by a particular system because it finds it to be the most efficient way for them to conduct their business. We have got to get to a point where we can build a relationship with communities so that the system reflects the kind of work that the people want to see done in their community. The boundaries, the populations, the priorities that the community sees are the ones that we're addressing with the public dollar. I think we've divided this country up in so many ways that people don't understand who the human service recipient is. When I go out to dinner with friends, and they say, "Oh, you're doing all that work for the poor," I say to them, "You know what? Human services, the public tax dollar touches you every day. You walk on it, you send your kids to it, every aspect of your life is touched by that public dollar and by the work that we do." We need to begin to have people form a relationship with that work. I think that we can benefit by looking at some of the models in entrepreneurial programs, when you have business executives working with young people and establishing some kind of mentoring relationship. We need to begin to do more of that. Bringing people together who don't necessarily see themselves as alike, beginning to work on the same kinds of problems and being able to find real solutions. But I think they need to see themselves as valuable resources. We've divided them up way too often.

Linda: There are very few examples of community-based health-care built on plans developed by residents of local areas. One way to judge whether the community members are involved in the health system is to look at governing structures of health systems. They're run by boards which rarely have significant consumer representation. The grievance structures are also indicative of the relationships with community members. If indeed a primary health care facility really is a community-based facility, users should have the ability to complain. Consumer representation should be an element in some aspect of how services are designed and delivered so that if something's wrong, grievances can be taken into account.

I'd like to say a couple of uplifting things. I work for a federally qualified health center which by law has to have a community-based board. I've enjoyed working in such an agency because it is governed by such a board. As a model, I would recommend looking at these boards to see where that leadership has come from and what people have done before they made so bold a move as to run a community-based health center. The other place I would look for good models is in birthing centers in other states which have been created through consumer-driven movements.

Gloria: The W. K. Kellogg Foundation has been engaged for the last several years in developing community-based primary health care models. When we talk about community-based, it is within the context of the community coming together to define who they are and what they are proposing to do to develop a healthy community. The perspective includes a continuum of services as well as looking at housing, safety of neighborhoods, job opportunities, and adequate nutrition. Many of the models were directed by nurses with several integrated into (and/or sustained by) larger organizations.

Question: In a focus on community-based programs, what is necessary in order to have both engagement and interaction among the key stakeholders?

Gloria: A major detriment for community participants to engaging and facilitating interaction among key stakeholders in community-based programming has to do with the time of meetings. They are usually held during the day when community residents are working and unable to attend. The first things to examine are when and where the meetings are scheduled and located. Are they held in the neighborhood, in the community, or is it expected that they travel a long distance? Is babysitting available? Another aspect apart from logistics is the importance of having a common vision with guiding principles so that all stakeholders feel a commitment to it.

Sibyl: We recently began to require that people who apply for grants from the Chicago Department of Public Health demonstrate a commitment to work with other providers in the community. We have nine clinics that provide health services. We have facility boards which consist of consumers from that particular region as well as other providers who live in that area. We found that their input and involvement have been very beneficial because many times people in the community have another perspective that we may not see.

Julio: Collaboration is a difficult thing because we ignore the fact that we are a diverse society with values that are very different from each other. I am a Latino male. My value system is very different from some of the people on this panel. I define "family" differently. I define "need" differently. We can't pretend that the values that I bring to the table don't guide the decisions that I make. We need to engage in a very difficult dialogue around our differences, but an even harder dialogue is around our values. How do we determine which values set the standards for the kind of work that we want to do? No amount of money is going to make that dialogue easier. It's being able to come to the table and say, "It doesn't matter how much money there is, because the work needs to be done."

Question: What lessons have you learned over time about how to sustain a program?

Linda: Would anyone in this room want to develop a five-year plan for a community-based provider system? The environment is mercurial. These systems must be prepared to be able to cross-subsidize their programs and to be able to sense trends in funding and respond to them.

Julio: In terms of sustaining a program, I would agree with you. I'm not sure, given the current climate, whether there's a really easy answer to that. We need to determine, "What are the outcomes, and how real are they for the people that they serve? Do they really meet what they perceive are their needs?" We have to define the system of care differently than it has been defined in the past. I think we have to be really clear about what the outcomes are for our investment. That's what will sustain effective programs in the future.

Sibyl: Dr. W. Edwards Deming is quoted as saying, "In God We Trust: All others must have data." When you see what the trends are, you really have to demonstrate the need for projects and show that need in terms of evaluation. Programs also have to demonstrate that they can be self supporting. We can no longer look to other people to fund the things that supposedly we should be interested enough in to make happen ourselves. Lastly, I think it's important for agencies to have someone to do their evaluation, someone to do their proposal, and someone to do their training. So I think that it's important to have someone who's on board who has the time and expertise to do the research required to apply for specific funding.

Gloria: I think there are different levels of sustainability that range from obtaining ongoing funds to continue the program to institutionalization of a model or curriculum within a larger organization. An example of the latter occurs when a university curriculum has moved from a clinical aspect to community based, and while that particular project may not have continued, the curriculum is integrated and becomes part of the educational process for healthcare professionals. I think in the arena of limited resources it is somewhat more challenging to obtain ongoing funds to sustain new organizations.

In the process of grant making in community-based programming, one of the lessons we've learned is the need to examine ways to build in economic development opportunities. How can we help communities look at their assets, strengths, and skills as a way to develop something that will help them economically?

Capacity building is another tool for assisting projects to sustain their efforts such as leadership development that takes into consideration convening and running meetings, grant writing, selection of board members and board training, application for 501(c)3 status, and the development of coalitions, to name a few.

Mary: You have to be prepared to have a prolonged period of high-risk investment and fund quite lavishly on faith for a time. If you're funding a new project, you've got to be there over time and invest quite substantially. You've got to think from the start about where the sustainable revenue stream is going to come from. There is plenty of money out there. It's simply a question of how we make decisions about how to deploy it within the total economy.

One success story was a program that created a "unified service plan" for a very high-risk, chronic mentally ill population in one of Chicago's suburban areas. This grant proposal came with a two-year timetable: The first six months involved hiring staff and planning the actual program. The second six months was a pilot phase during which the staff planned to take discharged patients from mental hospitals and then try to maintain them in a community with this unified service plan. And then there was a year scheduled in which they were going to operate the program.

As a program officer reviewing their first-year progress report, I was horrified to find that they had focused three staff people over a six-month period on six patients. This was appalling! How could one use this amount of resources and only deal with six people? It turned out that the staff deliberately chose six case examples of the most difficult types and conditions. They developed very good individual plans, worked at the case management and made it work. Subsequently, during their implementation year they increased their case loads to meet their stated numerical goals, and they did superbly.

They requested a third year of funding which was granted because "all the glitches weren't out of the system." At the end of that three-year period, this suburban authority went to its community and raised the tax rate to support the program which exists to this day. A program officer does not often have a story like that to tell. But it can happen, and I think that's how you build sustainable programs. You look to where the revenue stream is going to be, because foundation funding—and even government demonstration programs—are not going to be there over the long haul.

Question: What's the most pressing community-based health issue that we need to deal with?

Linda: I have two answers. One: As we all know, the determinants of health are not related to personal healthcare services. We need to look at what those determinants of "health" are and use those as the levers of control on which we build programs. Two: In the area of primary health care delivery, I think the most pressing problem is the growing number of uninsured citizens. We must reconsider what we have as a health system for delivery of personal health-care services and think about why we have the system we currently have. To me, a single-payer system appears to be the only mechanism for these sorts of changes.

Julio: The issue of economic development is a big one. We have got to begin to think about the role of economic development as it relates to healthcare. One: In terms of the environment that it creates. Two: The opportunity that either it does or doesn't present in terms of people being able to afford healthcare. And then my own bias, we can't have a country that ignores a good segment of its population because they are not legal residents. We cannot pretend that their health-care needs will somehow disappear just because they are no longer part of legislation.

Question: Are demonstration projects consistent with the notion of creating partnerships? When universities go out into neighborhoods, the community wants to know, "How long are you going to be here with us? Are you going to be here after your funding period, or are you just going to disappear in two years?"

Gloria: One of the things that I look at when I make a site visit to a prospective grantee is how the university views the com-munity and the community's perspective of the university. Is there talk about the community? Partnership? Collabo-ration? What is the university's past record with the com-munity? How often does the university go out to the community and actually walk and talk with the people?

I think the relationship goes way beyond sustaining a project. It begins long before a proposal is considered. Community/university partnerships are new ground for both, but especially for universities. They struggle as they learn these new paths to practice. There is a lot of work to be done prior to establishing a partnership. I am encour-aged by the efforts of the grantees that have entered into these relationships and by their commitment to the work they have undertaken.

Julio: I want to address this question because I think it's relevant to what we're trying to do in Illinois. It's monumental; it has tremendous possibilities for how we will do things in the future, not just in Illinois, but across the country. I'm part of a consortium of states, Michigan being one of them, that is really looking at how we are reinvesting our dollars, and it's not just healthcare. This is the Public Aid dollar, the Child Welfare dollar. What we did in the process of trying to look at "how do we reform the public system along with it's private providers" was to say, "This is a zero fund game. We're not going to give you new money to go off and create something." We said, "Look at the money that you currently have and think about how you would do something differently." When we talk about sustainability, you have to look at the dollars that are already there. The dollars that have already been invested. And to begin to think about how to create a partnership that meets everyone's agenda, that looks at the capacity at the table, and begins to think about where the gaps are. What is the role of the university? Is the data that universities create understandable by communities? I'll tell you from my experiences at this point: No. Not necessarily by any fault of their own, but they've been asking the wrong kinds of questions because they've been talking to themselves.

I want to use a really key example here. When I was working in Pilsen and Little Village (communities adjacent to this university) the number one problem they identified was rodent control. They said, "I don't care what you do around anything else, but if we're going to really deal with issues associated with children and health, we've got to get the city to do something about rats." It took four years and a program that came out of Community Policing for somebody to realize that was an issue, and you know what? A whole lot of healthcare problems got resolved because they dealt with the rat problem. This is significant. It's a new way of thinking, but we have to look at the current system and the resources we have. We've got to tap into the purse that's already there, because that's where the money is to sustain what we're going to be doing in the future. The money's there to create what we want, we just have to start to leverage it better.

Predictably, the views presented during this panel occurred along established "party lines," vis-a-vis funders, health professionals, and government officials. While acknowledging these diverse perspectives, perhaps the real value of these types of interactions comes from identifying the issues everyone seemed to agree on, such as:

- Many expound upon the importance of "community involvement" but few take the necessary (albeit difficult) steps to bring the consumer of the proposed service to the table as a meaningful stakeholder.
- For effective public/private partnerships to occur, incentives for all stakeholders must be provided, realistic goals must be set and agreed upon, and basic terminology must be clearly defined.
- While there is general recognition of this "new era of healthcare funding," there is still far too little consideration given to sustainability issues.

THE PANELISTS (ALPHABETICALLY)

Ada Mary Gugenheim

Program officer with principal responsibility for health programs of the Chicago Community Trust, a community foundation established in 1915 for the benefit of the residents of the greater Chicago area. Among her many accomplishments, Ms. Gugenheim was responsible for launching and managing a $10 million initiative designed to find and test new and improved ways of delivering cost-effective healthcare to the medically indigent.

Sybil Massey

Director of Grants Management, the Chicago Department of Public Health (CDPH). Ms. Massey has also served in the capacity of direct service provider and program director with mental health, social services, and alcoholism and substance abuse programs managed by the CDPH. She also volunteers with several youth and Christian-based programs in the area of "street counseling," and in 1996 received the City of Chicago Kathy Osterman award which recognizes city employees who have made outstanding contributions.

Gloria T. Meert

Program Director of Health Programming for the W. K. Kellogg Foundation, which was established in 1930 to "help people help themselves through the practical application of knowledge and resources to improve their quality of life and that of future generations." Ms. Meert evaluates and recommends proposals for funding, administers projects, and carries out other grant-making activities in the field of health. In addition to programming responsibilities, she assists with coordination of health programming including networking meetings, screening requests for funding, organizing other health-related meetings, and preparing reports.

Julio Rodriguez

Director of Community Resources and Development, the Governor's Task Force on Human Services Reform. Mr. Rodriguez is responsible for providing consultation and technical assistance to five community pilot sites (federations) across the state of Illinois. He works closely with the membership and staff of each federation to develop new and innovative ways for the state to respond to community needs.

Linda Diamond Shapiro

Director, Program Planning and Policy, Sinai Family Health Centers, a federally qualified health center with an integrated network of seventeen community health centers in underserved, low-income Chicago neighborhoods. Ms. Shapiro has extensive experience in the design and management of health and human service programs and expertise in strategic and long-range planning, public affairs, and policy analysis.

REFERENCES

Walker, B. J. Getting engaged: Turning rhetoric to reality in human services reform. In *Lessons learned 3, Reflections on leadership from the Annie E. Casey Foundation's Children and Family Fellowship Program,* Annie E. Casey Foundation, 701 St. Paul St., Baltimore, MD 21202, Spring 1996.

———. Human services reform in Illinois: Turning rhetoric to reality. In *Human services coordination: Who cares?* Policy Brief Report #1, available from the Evaluation and Policy Information Center, North Central Regional Educational Laboratory, 1900 Spring Rd., #300, Oak Brook, IL 60521, 1996.

Chapter 3

The Training of Community Health Advocates for Urban U.S. Communities: A Program Evaluation

CASSIA SOARES
SUSAN M. SWIDER
BEVERLY J. MCELMURRY

This project was supported by: the University of Illinois at Chicago (UIC) College of Nursing; the Chicago Community Trust; the W. K. Kellogg Foundation; the Robert R. McCormick Charitable Trust; the City of Chicago Mayor's Office of Employment and Training; the City of Chicago Department of Public Health; the Illinois Department of Transportation; and the U.S. Department of Health and Human Services, Office of Minority Health. At the time the training evaluation was conducted, Ms. Soares was a UIC graduate student, and Dr. Swider was coordinating the Primary Health Care in Urban Communities project, of which Dr. McElmurry was program director.

INTRODUCTION AND BACKGROUND

This chapter presents findings of the evaluation of a training program for community health advocates (CHAs) in an urban U.S. setting. These workers were trained in a university-based program developed by faculty and staff at the College of Nursing, University of Illinois at Chicago, over the period from 1987 to 1992. The training was part of a larger effort, the Primary Health Care in Urban Communities Project (PHCUC), developed to link health professionals, universities, and community residents together in coordinated efforts to identify and address community health concerns in selected inner-city neighborhoods (McElmurry et al., 1990; Swider & McElmurry, 1992).

The PHCUC project used the primary health care approach to achieve Health for All (WHO, 1978) with a special emphasis on community development. The community development approach to health planning views health as an outgrowth of the combined social, political, and economic conditions of individuals and communities. Health improvement is seen as a response to better living conditions, brought about by social and community action to change structural and environmental conditions, as well as changes in individual behavior. This approach is based on the assumption that community members can develop, by education and other means, the awareness and skills necessary to begin to take control of their health, and that improved community health will result from community involvement in health and development activities (Haglund, 1988).

Based on this, all PHCUC project components emphasized: collaboration between health professionals and community residents to achieve mutually agreed upon goals and activities; education and development activities for all participants; and a broad view of community health, encompassing economic, social, political, and cultural factors. After an initial training for the CHAs and health professionals, teams of nurses and CHAs worked in several community demonstration sites to identify and address neighborhood health concerns. In addition, other health professionals and CHAs participated in the training exercises and worked with other community organizations loosely affiliated with the PHCUC project. Over the five-year period of the project, over one hundred CHAs and more than two hundred health professionals participated in the project.

DESCRIPTION OF ADVOCATE TRAINING

Training Philosophy

The role of the CHA, as defined by the PHCUC project staff, was to work in their community to determine the residents' perceptions of their health and social needs; to provide health education and information to their neighbors; and to organize their neighbors to take collective action to address community health needs. Thus, the CHAs were seen as change agents who focus on health issues within their communities.

The training curriculum was built on a PHC/community health and development framework. In addition, teaching methods drew from the literature on adult education and the work of the Brazilian educator Paulo Freire. Freire (1970) stressed the importance of education for critical consciousness: that is, an ability to question the reality in which one lives and the underlying causes of that reality. This critical consciousness is requisite to becoming a change agent. Such education is focused on critical thinking and action based on reflection by the participants. Thus, the elements of community development, PHC, and education for critical consciousness are the underlying themes of the training philosophy. This philosophy is summarized in the following principles:

a. Health is seen in the context of life, as overall well-being, as opposed to the absence of disease or the simple delivery of services;
b. Social, political, cultural, and economic events and interactions affect and shape the health of the people;
c. Human beings are basically creative, rational, and analytical;
d. It is necessary to incorporate the ways of thinking and life experiences of the trainees in the training process;
e. Open dialogue during the teaching/learning process is fundamental; being willing to learn with others is essential;
f. Constant reflection is essential to critical thinking;
g. The idea of collaboration to solve problems and carry out goals is fundamental;
h. Commitment to addressing the health concerns expressed by people where they live and work is essential;
i. The knowledge exchange between instructors and trainees enriches the process of analysis of the lived experience and the development of critical thinking skills;
j. The starting point in learning is the previous knowledge the trainees have about any topic.

Training Goals

The overall goals of the training program were as follows:

1. Trainees would increase their knowledge of health and development issues in their communities;
2. The training session would encourage maximum participation on the part of the adult learners, with particular emphasis on incorporating the lived experience and previous knowledge of the trainees;
3. Successful participation in the training session would help to increase the critical thinking skills and problem-solving abilities of the trainees;
4. The trainees would complete the training session with an understanding of the role of a CHA in working to improve the health and development of their community.

Trainee Selection

The literature on CHWs strongly supports having such workers selected by and for the community in which they live, as a means of maximizing their ability to influence change among their neighbors (Swider & McElmurry, 1992). The PHCUC project operationalized this approach by relying on community organizations to recommend candidates for the training. These candidates had to meet minimum requirements of high school education or GED; residence in the community; expressed interest in community health or other community development activities; and being bilingual in communities where this was appropriate.

Over the five-year period of the project, 101 people were trained during seven different training periods for work in more than one dozen different communities in Chicago. Trainees were primarily female; African American (59%), Latino (37%), and other ethnic groups (4%), primarily Korean American.

Training Program Content

The training program focused on the health concerns of the trainees' communities and the role of a CHA in their neighborhood. The literature on CHA training documents the need for interactive learning methods; demonstration and sufficient practice time for any new skills acquired; and development of critical thinking and skills for working with people and systems within communities (Swider & McElmurry, 1992).

In light of the PHCUC philosophy about health and development, the training content was geared toward a broad view of health. Content included such topics as nutrition, housing, environmental health issues, parenting, communicable diseases, family planning, substance abuse, poverty and health, family violence, stress management, first aid, street safety, community organizing, and public aid (Swider & McElmurry, 1990). In addition, almost half of the training period was spent in field work in the communities with nurses and other CHAs to practice problem-solving skills, refine critical thinking abilities, and familiarize themselves with their new role in their neighborhood.

During the five years of the project, each of the seven training sessions for CHAs were conducted over a six-week period. Each six-week training session included 100 content hours and over 70 hours of community field experience. The classroom content was coordinated by project staff and taught by a variety of people, including experienced CHAs, community organizers, and university faculty from nursing, medicine, allied health, public health, and dentistry. Over time, the project staff implemented an orientation session for training faculty to help familiarize them with the training in its totality, understand the philosophy of the training, and begin to organize their material in light of the training philosophy. This orientation consisted of a two-hour session discussing the training program; brief comments on effective teaching methods for this population from faculty who had participated in the past; and a question-and-answer session.

EVALUATION OF PROGRAM

Evaluation Questions

The evaluation of the training program evolved over the five-year project period. That is, initial evaluation involved pre- and post-tests to measure changes in trainees' knowledge of training content. In the last training session, a fuller evaluation of the process of training and the training program's success in empowering trainees was conducted by the first author. The following questions guided the evaluation process:

1. Did the training session increase trainees' knowledge of health and development issues in their communities?
2. Did trainees participate in the training session and did their willingness and ability to participate increase over time?
3. Did the training sessions address the knowledge and lived experiences of the trainees?
4. Did the training session increase trainees' critical thinking skills?
5. Did the trainees gain an appreciation and understanding of their role as CHAs during the training session?

Evaluation Method

Prior to the evaluation discussed in this manuscript, the training sessions evaluation had focused on the knowledge gained by the trainees. The focus of the training, however, was broader than knowledge acquisition, and the project staff identified additional methods to evaluate the success of the broader program goals and philosophy. In the last training session of the five-year project period, the authors worked to develop a plan that evaluated trainees' development of a community empowerment philosophy.

Trainee Knowledge

The first part of the evaluation was focused on trainee knowledge acquisition, in response to evaluation question 1. This was measured via a pre- and post-test session for each six-week training segment. The questionnaire comprised of approximately fifty questions, was designed by faculty teaching the various content areas, to measure gain in knowledge for the trainees. Pre-and post-test data were collected for five of the seven training sessions, on a total of 73 trainees.

Training Process

To assess the training for participant teaching/learning interactions and the ability of the CHAs to improve critical thinking, a qualitative evaluation methodology was designed for the final six-week training session of the project. This session had 17 trainees (3 of Korean descent, 7 Latinos, and 7 African Americans). The training faculty teaching this session included project staff

(56%), university faculty (29%), and community leaders/activists (15%). Several instruments were developed to assess the interactive teaching/learning process and gather in-depth, detailed data focusing on the trainees' reactions to, and perceptions of, the training process. The data were collected via observations of the training session and a focus group session conducted on the last day of the session.

Session Observations

Observations of the training classes in the last training session were conducted to address evaluation questions 2, 3, and 4. The training class observations were conducted by the first author functioning as a participant/observer, under the generally accepted rule of not changing the normal development of the sessions (Patton, 1975). In this role, the evaluator clarified classroom issues when it seemed appropriate and assisted with the structural and operational development of the classes (e.g., distributing materials to the trainees). This evaluator developed a positive rapport with the trainees, who included her in their comments and requested her participation in role-playing activities. This level of trust helped to foster deeper discussions and encouraged trainees to feel free to express ideas and criticisms among each other and between trainee and instructor.

The observations took place during the entire six-week training session, with a focus on trainee/faculty interactions for the observations. The evaluator reviewed all written project materials (goals, philosophy, conceptual framework, evaluation plan) and then observed three training classes. She then used this information to design a class observation form that was further refined during use at the next four sessions. On the observation form, the evaluator responded to thirteen questions that asked about advocates' participation in the sessions. In addition to rating overall class participation and mood (e.g., 5 = attentive; 1 = bored), and rate of talk during the session, the evaluator noted whether the instructor requested trainees to participate in the session, asked them for examples from their own lives, used real life situations to develop concepts, used visual aids, and included trainees in the development of the class. Directly addressing trainees' behavior, other questions asked whether the trainees could hear and easily understand what the instructor was saying; whether they were taking the initiative to give examples from their own lives; and whether interaction between trainees and instructor changed over the individual session. The final question asked about evidence of critical thinking skills which here are generally classified into five types: (1) breaking silence, (2) adding to a discussion to clarify or ask questions, (3) giving ideas, (4) summarizing or conceptualizing, and (5) critically evaluating ideas or calling for solutions. The evaluator completed a different form, consisting of three questions, after the session ended. These questions asked whether the underlying philosophical themes of the training program were being addressed by each session; whether the session was characterized by a feeling of exchange and sharing among class participants; and whether the instructor seemed more interested in addressing the needs of the class or covering the session's content.

Entire sessions were observed, and each lasted one to three hours. The evaluator collected data for 41 of the 44 training sessions conducted (95%). The evaluator also audiotaped all training classes, listened to each tape, and collected appropriate data using the post-session guide.

This responsive and formative evaluation was designed to be consistent with the project goals, and it helped the evaluator gain a better understanding of the training process over time. She analyzed data for questions and themes that emerged and changed throughout the training session (Shadish et al., 1991). In addition, another member of the project staff observed one training class using the session observation guide to check inter-rater reliability and to minimize bias in data collection and interpretation.

Focus Group

At the completion of the entire six-week training session, the evaluator conducted a focus group with the trainees to elicit their perceptions of their role as CHAs; their views of health within the general structure of society; and their views of the overall training program, to address evaluation question 5 (Appendix A). The authors thought a focus group would be a useful technique to answer these evaluation questions because of the proven utility of this method to elicit feedback from small groups of people in a supportive, respectful climate (Basch, 1987; Ramirez & Sheppard, 1988).

DATA ANALYSIS AND RESULTS

Evaluation Question 1:   Did the training session increase trainees' knowledge of health and development issues in their communities?

The quantitative evaluation of knowledge gained by the trainees over the training period was conducted with five of the seven groups of trainees. The post-test scores were significantly higher than the pre-test scores (paired t-value = 6.43, n = 73, p < .0001). Thus, trainees did leave the training session with increased health and development knowledge, consistently, over the five-year project period.

Evaluation Question 2:   Did trainees participate in the training session and did their willingness and ability to participate increase over time?

The classroom observation tool was used to document trainee participation during the last training session of the project. Using this guide, the evaluator documented whether and how the trainees were encouraged to participate during the training. The instructors' requests for trainee participation occurred in many different ways. The majority of the sessions used the strategy of question/answer between instructors and trainees. Those questions that received the most participation from the trainees were those that the trainees could relate to their background and experience. For example, all the trainees who were parents eagerly responded to such questions as: "Have you ever had an experience with a doctor who did not completely examine a child?" or "What do we want for our children?" Trainee-to-instructor questioning occurred during the sessions and was sometimes encouraged at the end.

Questions perceived as "foreign," too complex, or too technical for the trainees' backgrounds brought confusion, tension, and silence. For example, the question, "What makes HIV epidemiologically difficult to trace?" paralyzed the class and prompted the instructor to break the question down into simpler parts before proceeding. Other questions were asked at inappropriate moments. For example, expecting conceptual understanding at the start of a class can be problematic, for example, "When you are in a good health state, what is your expected behavior?" Role-playing activities were also used during a few training classes to complement the trainees' comprehension of an issue (e.g., to illustrate a discussion session about necessary skills for health advocates).

The use of a variety of teachers sometimes resulted in missed opportunities to help trainees make connections between topics. For example, in a class on community organizing, the discussion and role-playing were each conducted by a different instructor. The discussion session addressed advocates' roles in community meetings, the interplay of teaching and learning with neighbors, and positive advocate/community relations. The role-playing session explored confrontation between people and governmental officials. Both classes were productive in terms of participation, but the connection between the two related classes was never developed. For the most part, however, participation was nurtured in many different ways. The most productive and resourceful techniques for facilitating participation were role playing, problem solving; open discussion, and warm-up/sensitization games.

The importance of using everyday life experiences of the learners (trainees) in an educational dialogue about concrete issues and problems is stressed in the adult education literature (Freire, 1970). However, the instructor must differentiate between types of life situations. For example, it is qualitatively different to elicit trainee comments about how embarrassing it is for a teen to buy condoms in public places than to elicit comments on a patient's resistance to a therapeutic regime and his/her need to change medications to be cured. The first example is readily understandable; it pertains to most people's lives and therefore can be used to develop critical thinking processes. The second example is information, and while it assists the learner in understanding the technical skills of healthcare providers, it does not take advantage of the trainees' experiences to explore and analyze their perceptions.

Evaluation Question 3:   Did the training sessions address the knowledge and lived experiences of the trainees?

The observations of classroom interactions also focused on whether the trainees were encouraged to give examples from their lives in class. While trainees often shared their lived experiences, this happened at their own initiative much more often than as a result of instructor encouragement. Trainees shared many significant experiences about their mistreatment in governmental offices, diseases of relatives and friends, stories about their children's behavior, personal domestic violence experiences, and language difficulties. However, in observing how the instructors treated such information, the evaluator observed that most such remarks were usually acknowledged respectfully, but rarely used by the instructors to explore a new idea or spontaneously alter the course of a class. One example of building content around the lived experience was an instructor's response to a trainee comment that her children became willing to feed themselves at a certain age. The instructor used this as a springboard to discuss development of autonomy in children. This response valued the trainee experience and constituted an effort to construct a concept using the trainee's knowledge. However, this example was the exception rather than the rule.

The practice of incorporation of the lived experiences of the learners into the classroom could have also been used to model the role of community educator that CHAs would use in their later work. However, on the contrary, there were times when the instructor refocused a lively discussion, for example, on immigration and naturalization, to pursue a planned emphasis on problem-solving strategies, thereby addressing one set of trainee expectations while stifling interesting discourse.

The most common instructor response to trainee experiences was a passive incorporation of the remarks, demonstrated by such statements as "That is OK," or "That can happen," which simply validates a given situation without taking the opportunity to explore it. For example, when an instructor comments that the high rate of teenage pregnancies is sad, she communicates the inevitability of the situation and ignores the consciousness-raising opportunity to discuss the cycle of related issues, such as poverty, frustration, self-esteem, and contraceptive technology.

Throughout the training, the need to build on trainees' existing knowledge base and communicate appropriately was expressed by trainees. Sessions were evaluated in terms of language appropriateness, comprehensibility of the material, use of colloquial and metaphoric expressions, and use of complicated concepts. While expressions such as "degenerative nature," "randomized studies," "cell vulnerability," "psychological function," "herd immunity," and "residues from stroke," were used by instructors accustomed to speaking in an academic setting, the instructors often tried to make expressions and/or technical language easily accessible. This attitude improved communication and contributed to the dialogue by engaging everyone in solving certain mysteries of the English language. Some language problems did not disturb the learning process, when either the instructor or the trainees took the initiative to resolve the problem. The classes that did not overcome the communication problem were the ones in which other interactive dynamics were also problematic.

Other class techniques nurtured feelings of sharing among class participants. For example, when instructors shared their personal feelings and experiences and/or encouraged feelings of complicity, they opened the door to group dialogue and interaction. When the trainees identified with other people's experiences, they felt secure in talking about their own experiences. When the instructor's attitude fostered participation and instructor and trainees allowed each other the necessary time to formulate their ideas, the distance between them diminished. As the goal of this training was not quantity but rather quality of information, it was not necessary for instructors to conclude "There is no time!" or "We have to cover too much material!" In participatory education, the instructor must make the shift from "speaking to" to "speaking with." Advocates were being trained for community leadership and this leadership needed to be demonstrated. These ideas were incorporated to some extent by the project staff and by some of the community activists who came to teach classes, but tended to be used less by those with academic or clinical backgrounds. Of course there were exceptions, that is, some instructors from academic settings who established effective dialogue and some from community organizations who did not.

One common tendency among instructors was to favor themes they deemed likely to generate fruitful dialogue because they had worked in the past or tapped into trainees' day-to-day experience. In either case, such a bias reinforced the artificial distance between academic (knowledge) and community life (experience). Conversely, the routine problems in the community, such as housing and public aid, were often fertile topics for lively class discussion due to the trainees' familiarity with the problems and the instructors' convictions about the topic's relevance. Educators will favor strategies involving dialogue only when they believe rapport can be successfully established. Otherwise, they tend to opt for the traditional kind of session—a lecture. Particularly in technical sessions such as anatomy or sexually transmitted diseases, the tendency was to use a clinical approach. However, in a session on AIDS the use of warm-up and sensitization exercises succeeded in fostering intense dialogue, a sharing climate and productive discussion.

One problem was the tendency for instructors to focus on covering class content rather than meeting the expressed needs of the participants. Thus, we evaluated the overall interest of faculty in covering the session contents and addressing the needs of the class. Twenty-nine of the forty-one observed sessions were scored in this way, with a rank of 1 = addressing class needs and 5 = covering session content. Only 21 percent of the observed sessions were ranked 1 or 2, indicating a need for stronger efforts to address expressed class needs. In other instances, trainees did not participate and therefore their needs, though clearly not compatible with what was being presented, remained unspoken. Trainees at times indicated boredom by reading newspapers or talking with colleagues, or in some cases indicating that they did not understand what the instructor was saying. These appeared to be trainee attempts to change the course of the session.

One problematic tendency observed was for instructors to slacken on their teaching responsibilities in the name of interactive learning. Such behavior took different forms, such as not preparing for sessions, relying too heavily on improvisation, arriving late or even missing sessions. Instructor absence or tardiness occurred approximately 10 percent of the time. This modeled irresponsible behavior and absenteeism among trainees. Instructors generally had to wait a few minutes to start the class due to tardiness among the trainees. This appeared to be caused more by the lack of support in the trainees' personal lives than by an environment of permissibility. Among those trainees who received monetary compensation for the training, the absenteeism for the observed sessions was around 5 percent.

Twenty-nine of the forty-one observed class sessions were ranked for overall trainee participation and on a scale of 1 = bored or distracted to 5 = attentive, 66 percent of these sessions received an overall rank of 4 or 5.

Evaluation Question 4:   Did the training session increase trainees' critical thinking skills?

Results of the observational data were classified into five categories of increasing levels of critical thinking.

1. Breaking silence or tension, answering simple questions.
This category included such comments as "Drugs must be expensive," referring to a teenager's ability to acquire drugs, or "I love chocolate," in a discussion about healthy habits. Such comments do not necessarily involve interaction but are attempts to participate. Also included in this category were direct answers to simple questions.

2. Adding to the discussion to clarify or ask questions.
This category exemplified the willingness to ask questions, a more complex form of participation requiring more attention and explanation. Examples of this included: "Why don't we breastfeed in this country?" when discussing the advantages of breastfeeding, or "She is an expert in breastfeeding," indicating why one colleague's statement should be valued.

3. Giving ideas, examples from their lives that fit the discussion.
This level of participation requires comfort in talking about personal experiences and being secure that one's statement will be appropriate to the class. Examples include, "In Mexico, we take the BCG vaccination; my PPD here was positive because of that," during a discussion about tuberculosis in the United States; or "Once a homeless lady came to my door at two in the morning to ask for help," referring to problems which come with being a health advocate in the community.

4. Summarizing, conceptualizing, establishing links and correlations.
Examples are: "If you have AIDS and you do not have any kind of support system for AIDS, you get depressed and you get sicker," agreeing with the instructor about the need for a support system for AIDS patients. Or, "This

year, because of the cuts in public aid, we are going to see many more homeless people out there," during a discussion about the present situation of subsidized housing.

5. Evaluating ideas critically and calling for solutions.
This category is distinguished from the preceding one by including proposals for action and solutions. "Because my mother raised me with the right to discuss at home, I feel comfortable and I know I have the right to express my opinions and that is the way it should be for everyone," referring to how communication happens in society and its social and cultural influences. Or, "Every time my son had to pay for lunch, the teacher would keep the change. I realized this was not right and I called the principal and asked about it. If this had not worked, I would call the other parents and take other actions," referring to the process of organizing and mobilizing for rights in society.

Such categories inevitably overlapped. Some trainees cited examples from their own lives and also called for solutions. Nevertheless, some interesting patterns emerged. Categories 1–3 were the most often seen, indicating a strong level of participation in relation to a weak process of critical elaboration. The frequency of remarks in the last two categories increased somewhat during the second half of the training, indicating a positive evolution of critical thinking. These latter sessions were also the ones in which instructors clearly used discussion as a classroom strategy, allowing the thought processes to develop. Furthermore, those trainees who demonstrated the ability to make more incisive remarks did so right from the beginning of the training, and they improved slightly over time. A small group of trainees increased their critical thinking abilities during the second half of the training. For the first three categories, the pattern of participation increased more over the training than for the last two categories.

Evaluation Question 5:   Did the trainees gain an appreciation and understanding of their role as CHAs during the training session?

The focus group was designed to elicit trainee opinions of the training program. We particularly wanted to evaluate whether the training method stimulated a participatory process, awakened their perceptions of health within the general structure of society, and assisted them to envision and operationalize their role as a CHA.

After explaining the focus group objectives and the importance of their feedback, the trainees were provided a piece of blank unlined paper and colored markers. They were asked to first draw pictures representing the experience for them and then explain their pictures to the rest of the group. This activity was extremely fruitful; participation was intense as the trainees enthusiastically disclosed their personal views and thoughtful insights. The discussion was entirely dominated by the trainees and the moderator role was confined to organization of time, sequential introduction of issues according to the suggested guide, and encouraging a balance in participation.

The drawings were analyzed or "decodified" in a Freirian framework and interpreted. There were two major patterns exhibited among the many qualities displayed.

1. The Change Pattern.
This was illustrated by drawings showing training as an educational "door" to a better life for the advocate and community; or a drawing depicting the advocates' shift in focus and priority from her home to her community (Figure 1).

2. The Acquisition Pattern.
This was depicted by drawings showing trainees acquiring knowledge, strength, and new friends during the training period (Figure 2).

In the subsequent discussions, criticisms of the class sessions were related to an excess of technical information, especially about HIV and STDs. Some trainees described "numbers" as difficult to grasp and not important to the content. Some instructors were criticized for being unable to stimulate participation and therefore "losing" the class.

The trainees also concluded that they needed more discussion about general community problems such as housing and public aid, besides laws and means of access to the public health system. Therefore, more space should be dedicated to those issues, as well as to nutritional education, and less time devoted to health-disease technical information. The field experience and training manual were both favorably reviewed.

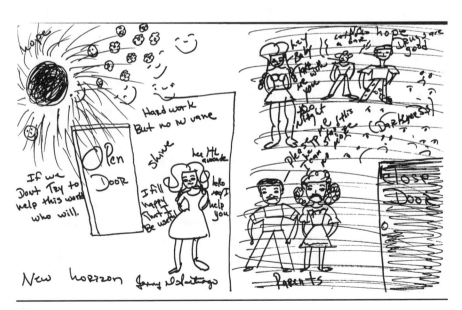

FIGURE 1.
Caption

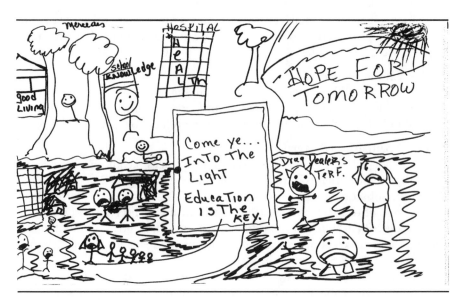

FIGURE 2.
Caption

CONCLUSIONS AND RECOMMENDATIONS

The training program for the CHAs was developed and revised over a number of years according to new insights in the field and constant informal evaluation. The evaluation described here was characterized by three assumptions:

1. A real dialogical process must be created to allow the exchange of experiences and knowledge among instructors, project members, and new trainees. This exchange can facilitate comprehension of the community reality and is necessary to undertaking any community development effort.
2. No education is ever neutral. The concepts expressed are not value neutral, that is, they represent a particular view of health and illnesses and their relation to social systems. This relationship can be expressed as a function of current society or as a critique of society as it relates to health and development.
3. Participation as an educational tool should accelerate the process of critical thinking and produce change. The institutionalized health educational process reproduces the same social reality when it charges the individual with the responsibility of adaptation to the way the system is designed. Here, we are referring to structural changes, those that are needed to transform the system and reflect the community needs.

Some important points that maximized the effects of these activities were pre-organization of the event in conjunction with, and as a complement to, other activities; coordination among instructors; intense participation of instructors;

establishment of clear examples and objectives, with written statements of the cases for role play; permanence of the same discussion groups; inclusion of all participants; design of small group assignments; and wrapping up to allow opportunity to critique and digest the process, so that references or conclusions do not get lost or forgotten.

When discussions drew on the trainees' own backgrounds and experiences, participation was excellent and fruitful, with high levels of critical thinking exhibited by the trainees. In general, however, the critical thinking process could be further stimulated in the training. The overall training objective is for the CHA to develop an ability to analyze issues in all spheres of life in order to comprehend social dynamics, relationships among social classes, causes of inequalities, and how these factors are related to community health and development. Health access issues need to be further explored, leading trainees to a more global comprehension of the social system and thereby raising their consciousness of the issues.

The process of questioning the causes of ill health in society that occurred during the training was not systematic. Open discussion of proposed themes and group participation in determining the pace and content of the classes should be stressed as a project methodology to teach community organizing skills. One example of this was a session which began with each trainee singing the national anthem of the country from which they came. A fruitful discussion ensued about different problems in different countries, interference of one country with another, and how these issues affect a population's health. According to Freire (1970), education for critical consciousness, that is, for questioning and challenging assumptions about oneself and one's society, stresses action-based reflection by the people. Application of this approach involves analyzing the perception of health and medical care within the total structure of society.

Open discussion of topics relevant to trainees' lives is a potential mechanism for achieving perception and participation in critical consciousness. Such discussion allows the group to creatively construct their thought processes and conclusions. The role of the instructor/facilitator is crucial to develop an atmosphere of participation and guiding discussion. When people are accustomed to consuming packaged information, they need time and assistance to construct new views. The task of the educator is to organize activities that counteract the lack of interest in social and political affairs, and that sharpen discussions and proposals for action (Lovett et al., 1983).

The relationship between academic and community people is important on two counts. First, the exchange of knowledge is a dialogical process. Without this process, or willingness to create it, conflicts persist and result in discussion instead of dialogue. In health education, individuals are charged with the responsibility for changing life styles in order to eliminate risk behaviors for disease. Yet change in personal behavior depends fundamentally on the availability of other support structures. Low-income community people often have limited money and unsatisfactory social supports; frequently their basic needs are unmet (Salmon, 1991). Second, the medicalization of symptoms that result from the social sources of distress and disease is often blamed on the victims as being due to their ideology or personal lifestyle (Kleinman, 1988).

Academic professionals involved with the CHA training must understand the philosophy of community development. Workshops for instructors provide a means to discuss the contents and methodology of training for development. To prepare CHAs for an active role in the transformation of society, instructors must have techniques for stimulating participation and critical thinking in order to help trainees focus on the search for underlying causes of problems and their consequences. Expertise and academic knowledge need not conflict with a realistic approach to the training of health advocates. Also, the above comments are valid for instructors from community organizations, even those who already practice educational methods suited to community development. One possibility is to develop a bibliography in this area that is made available as an instructor's manual.

Another idea for encouraging improved faculty/trainee interaction is to further develop the instructor orientation. Such development might include further discussion of the teaching/learning principles discussed here, with small group discussion and/or role playing of methods to address content and process. In addition, CHAs could be involved in these workshops and could even be paired with instructors to co-present training classes. This partnership would provide an opportunity for both the faculty and trainee to work closely and observe each other's teaching/learning styles. It would also provide the instructor with feedback on accessibility of content for the trainees. Such interaction would require a great deal of time and willingness, on the part of both the teacher and the trainee, to work at this process. Additional support for development of this training work would be helpful.

The above type of training offers an outstanding opportunity to use the views of academics, community activists, community residents, and health advocates. A balance of participants realizes consistency and diversity through the group's efforts to overcome discrepancies and discuss ideas. Discussions are important to improve a group's practical and technical information related to a given theme. It is important to use examples and practical activities to avoid sessions that overwhelm learners with abstract information. Such activities facilitate trainee participation even when discussing subjects of a technical nature. Anatomical information, for example, can be more stimulating when associated with health problems. The digestive system can be studied during the nutrition sessions, and the respiratory and cardiac systems during classes on heart disease. By using simple dough and paint, the trainees can sculpt and color their versions of internal organs and compare them with models. In fact, games and the use of the arts in general are an alternative to verbal and written communication and constitute an important health education training tool, especially in communities where literacy levels are low or where English is the second language of the participants.

The focus group revealed that the trainees liked the experience of mingling with people of different races and different nationalities. To some extent the experience resulted in a group identification not usually allowed by the geographic division of the population in this and other cities. It was a revelation to participants that many problems faced by low-income communities are similar. They found a powerful community organizing tool in being able to work together across ethnic and racial divisions. Individuals develop an understanding of their class situation in relation to others. It is also important to note at this point that the United States is the only major developed Western nation whose government does not collect mortality statistics by class. For the health fields, the study and interpretation of health problems are often based on racial analyses. Yet we know that the way people live, get sick, and die depends on their race, sex, age, and also on the socioeconomic class to which they belong (Navarro, 1991). It is fruitful for teachers and trainees alike to discuss class as a factor in health differences, as well as race/ethnicity.

In summary, the training described here is an excellent beginning to the process of developing mechanisms for collaboration between community residents and health professionals for improved mutual understanding and development as well as implementation of community health and development efforts in urban U.S. communities. The evaluation data and recommendations suggest ongoing revisions to the training process to better meet the overall health and development goals of the communities served by the health advocates.

REFERENCES

Basch, C. E. (1987). Focus group interview: An underutilized technique for improving theory and practice in health education. *Health Education Quarterly, 14,* 411–448.

Freire, P. (1970). The pedagogy of the oppressed. New York: Penguin.

Haglund, B. J. (1988). The community diagnosis concept—a theoretical framework for prevention in the health sector. *Scandinavian Journal of Primary Health Care,* Suppl. 1, 11–21.

Jarvis, P. (1983). *Adult and continuing education: Theory and practice.* London: Croom Helm.

Kleinman, A. (1988). *The illness narratives.* New York: Basic Books.

Lovett, T., Clarke, C. & Kilmurray, A. (1983). *Adult education and community action.* London: Croom Helm.

McElmurry, B. J., Swider, S. M., Bless, C., Murphy, D., Montgomery, A., Norr, K., Irvin, Y., Gantes, M. & Fisher, M. (1990). Community health advocacy: Primary health care nurse-advocate teams in urban communities. In National League for Nursing (Ed.), *Perspectives in nursing 1989–1991,* New York: NLN.

Navarro, V. (1991). Race or class or race and class: Growing mortality differentials in the United States. *International Journal of Health Services, 21,* 229–235.

Patton, M. Q. (1975). *Alternative evaluation research paradigm.* North Dakota: University of North Dakota Press.

Ramirez, A. Z. & Sheppard, J. (1988). The use of focus groups in health research. *Scandinavian Journal of Primary Health Care,* Suppl. 1, 81–90.

Salmon, J. W. (1991). Introduction of section on health promotion strategies. *International Journal of Health Services, 21,* 417–421.

Shadish, W. R., Cook, T. D. & Leviton, L. C. (1991). *Foundations of program evaluation.* California: Sage.

Swider, S. M. & McElmurry, B. J. (1990). A women's health perspective in primary health care: A nursing and community health worker demonstration project in urban America. *Journal of Family and Community Health, 13,* 1–17.

World Health Organization (1978). *Primary health care: The Alma Ata Declaration.* Switzerland: WHO.

APPENDIX A

Focus Group Evaluation Form
(Total time: 1–1.5 hours)

1. *Introduction* (5 minutes)

   Opening. Welcome everyone to activity; emphasize importance of session in terms of training improvement. Explain there are no right or wrong answers; interest is on the ideas, opinions, and concerns that they have been developing during the training.

   Mechanism. Arrange chairs in a circle. Point out that the tape recorder is a helper device. Remind trainees that their opinions will be treated confidentially. Have probe instructions written on a board to ensure understanding.

2. *Warm-up* (30 minutes)

   Generating pictures. (15 minutes) What is the training all about? What is the meaning of the training? Give all participants color markers and an unlined, blank paper large enough to be seen by everyone. Ask participants to draw a picture to represent the training, or what they consider significant or something that could summarize the main idea.

   De-codification process. (15 minutes) Give all participants a few minutes each to show their pictures and tell the group what their picture means and why they chose the picture.

3. *Discussion Guide* (50 minutes)

   After the above activity, moderator starts the discussion using the following questions:

   What are the factors that can affect your health?

   Among those, or others you can think about, what are the most important problems you can detect in your communities?

   Who has the responsibility for the health of the population?

   What are the actions that we can take to improve the health conditions?

   How do you see the role of the health advocate?

   How have you felt about in-class presentations? Include comments about level, quantity, and quality of material (including manual), etc.

   How have you felt about the training time in the community with the other advocates? Include problems and difficulties as well as suggestions.

Chapter 4

The Community Health Advocate's Point of View

KATHLEEN F. NORR
BEVERLY J. MCELMURRY
SUSAN J. MISNER

First and foremost, our thanks go to the many community health advocates who have worked with us throughout our various community outreach projects. To wit: Mary L. Bell, Lusita Collazo, Tasha Coursey, Carmen Flores, Willamette Douglas, Juana Gonzalez, Martha Gonzalez, Janice Hamilton, Nayda Hernandez, Ursula Hunt, Tamika Lee, Phillip Lewis, Karen Martin, Celia Martinez, Mary Owens, Vivian Price, Socorro Ramos, Mildred M. Rodriguez, Anniece Seymore, and Magnolia Whitaker. Finally, we are most appreciative of the funders and supporters of these projects who gave so willingly, so often. Our thanks go to the Chicago Community Trust, the W. K. Kellogg Foundation, the Robert Wood Johnson Foundation, the Chicago Department of Public Health, Blue Cross and Blue Shield, and (of course) the University of Illinois at Chicago College of Nursing.

The College of Nursing at the University of Illinois at Chicago has been involved for over ten years in implementing primary health care in the urban inner city through a nurse/advocate team model. Several chapters in this book describe how this model has been implemented through various projects as well as the role of advocates from the perspective of professional project directors. However, there is no description of the advocate role as seen from the inside, by the advocates themselves.

The conceptual model presented in the introductory chapter describes the nurse/advocate team, supported by university-based staff, as a way to link the community, healthcare system, and university in health promotion. We used this model as a framework for organizing and presenting the advocates' perspectives on their role, including its satisfactions and frustrations. Next, their views about the team are presented, including advocate-to-advocate, advocate-nurse, and advocate-to-university staff relationships. We then discuss how advocates view their community, university, and healthcare system, as well as possible solutions to community problems. Finally, the advocates discuss how their work changed their lives.

METHOD

Multiple qualitative data sources presenting the perspective of the advocates were integrated to develop the themes presented here. Initially, in-depth individual interviews were conducted with nine advocates who had been involved in the process for one to five years at the time of the interview in 1991. An interview guide was used that listed a set of themes or areas to be discussed, but the advocates were encouraged to expand upon these issues as they wished and to add any additional thoughts they had.

Later, focus groups provided a second major data source. After each training session was completed, a focus group was conducted with newly trained advocates to elicit their thoughts and feelings about the training process and how the experience had affected their lives. The discussion guide for this round of conversations focused on the advocates' training experience, their views of their communities and community health, their views and feelings about the advocate role based on their limited field experience during training, and how the training had affected them personally. Finally, in preparation for this book, eleven experienced health advocates (most of whom were still working in the field) were brought together for a reunion focus group in December 1996. This gathering focused on the advocate role in the community—its strengths, frustrations, and the concerns the participants may have had about their role.

All transcripts of focus groups and interviews were professionally transcribed and entered into the Ethnograph software package where themes were identified and coded.

RESULTS

How Advocates View their Role

In most primary health care (PHC) projects advocates do a wide variety of health promotion activities, such as problem solving with individual clients, offering group health promotion sessions, and networking with other organizations and agencies within and outside the community. (See Chapter 6, Evaluating PHC in Urban Communities, for a description of the number and variety of these different activities in one project.) There is no particular activity that advocates can claim as their sole area of expertise. Instead, the diverse combinations of advocate experiences makes the way they offer health promotion services different from either healthcare professionals or untrained community residents. Advocates bring to their job their life experience as members of the community they serve. They acquire health information through their initial and continuing training. Through their work as advocates they build a network of ties to other organizations within and outside their community. Integrating their life experiences, training, and organizational ties makes them effective role models, teachers, and bridges between community residents and other agencies and services.

Personal Experience

The advocates bring from the community an in-depth understanding of the situations residents face based on their personal experiences. This understanding establishes a common ground where they can meet residents as equals. In the words of one advocate:

> I notice one of the important things is the confidentiality that I've developed with them and they with me. That they're able to talk with me about things that they're afraid to tell other people, or come out and say them to anyone, period. . . . And I always make it clear to them that I'm not a social worker and that I don't criticize.

Living in the community gave the advocates unique access to people and areas not usually reached by health professionals and clinics. The advocates derived a great deal of satisfaction from being able to help their neighbors both formally on the job and informally at home. One advocate said, "Someday, I got to get my own blood pressure kit because a lot of people be coming to me, you know, who have elder grandmothers or mothers who want me to take their pressure. A lot of people's concerned about their blood pressure and cholesterol." Another advocate described how she found out about a neighbor's needs through her children:

> I knew that they were homeless. My children told me, so they brought the little boy over. So I told him, "You know, if your mom feels like

she needs to talk to me, she can." You know. So this is a neighborhood referral, you know, with children doing the work.

Shared lived experiences also make the advocates uniquely effective as role models. Unlike professionals, advocates can truly claim to have achieved the personal life changes they promote. One advocate described how her job led to discussions with her friends and neighbors about how they too might change their lives.

> Then I told them [about my job]. "Oh, you are not on public aid anymore?" And I said, "No, not intend to be all my life." Don't get me wrong. Public aid is nice, but it was meant to help you. Not to stick there. It is to help you to help yourself and otherwise. And we elaborated on those issues.

Advocates emphasize the personal choices their clients can make that will better enable them to do more for themselves. One advocate explained:

> They want to know how they can get out of the situation that they are in. Like that, you know? And then a black person, they feel like they are being bombarded, you know, and there is no way out. You know, like I told them that there is a way out, but you have to dig your way out. Education, think good about yourself, support groups, parent support groups, and things like that.

Another advocate said: "To let them know that they can get out of what they are in, that is my goal. . . . Just because you live in a place, you don't have to be a part of the problem. You can be a part of the solution."

Their shared experiences increase the validity of the advocates' counsel in the eyes of their neighbors, but it also creates a degree of stress for the advocates. Sometimes the advocate's success created jealousy on the part of former friends. As one advocate said: "Because once upon a time I used to be on public aid and now I'm not and a lot of them feel . . . you know how it is, you get a job, 'Ah! She thinks she's more than what's what.'" It is very difficult for the advocate not to become personally, emotionally involved in their cases. Frequently, listening to a client brings back memories of personal bad experiences, which distresses the advocate. One advocate recalls:

> You know, they'll break out and cry in front of us, and you see that and, sort of like, it makes you think. You sort of like get flashbacks of when you were caught up in a situation like that, or maybe you knew someone who was caught up in a situation like that, a family member, a friend, you know. You don't really want to sit there and cry with a client.

Sharing New Knowledge

The advocates acquire new knowledge from their training about health and education, and they find great personal satisfaction in sharing that information. One advocate said: "I was really like afraid of HIV and I didn't want to hear about it. But as I have learned, now I feel like I can teach people this. And I want to teach people this so they won't be scared like I was."

Another advocate observed how important health education can be:

> What I am thinking about in education is like the workshops that we
> do or like for the AIDS to tell them, "Hey. You can be protected."
> About a child, how can you tell if a child is really sick? Or how can you
> try to feed him better if you don't have enough money? If these
> people could get to all these things, then their life would be improved.

Advocates also found that education can make a difference. One advocate shared her views about parenting:

> I was telling them to remember to hug the children and sit down and
> find out what the child is trying to tell you, you know? Some moms is
> so quick to hit and call those other languages to their children, and
> you know, I told them that is not very healthy. Whatever you put into
> a kid, you are going to put back out. So they're beginning to notice a
> change in their children.

Advocates pointed out the importance of broad-based health knowledge for their jobs. One observed: "When we go out and we do presentations . . . it could be on one subject, but a hundred other subjects could come up. So that's why I think if you're a health advocate, you know, your role is many roles, not just one."

Advocates developed effective ways of integrating their new knowledge with their lived experiences. They are very sensitive to their audience's response and develop a sense of when they are connecting and communicating effectively. One advocate described her approach to health education:

> Looking at the house and how people react. When you know that they
> don't know nothing about what you're talking about and when they
> leave, they at least have a sense of what you've said. You know, if it was
> about family planning, about sexually transmitted diseases, about
> domestic violence, about stress. You know that they're leaving with
> some knowledge, a little knowledge about something.

Another advocate ascribed her popularity as an educator to the way she was able to communicate:

> You know, you get their attention, if you just calm yourself down,
> and knowing what you are going to give to them and help them

understand the information and you know, the literature that you've got. You know, you take it out and give some handouts and you just talk to them like . . . a mom to her daughters."

Often advocates are struggling to make the same health changes they are teaching, which gives a genuineness to their messages. "Sometimes I feel as though I am being hypocritical teaching nutrition, you know, but I found out that it is a process that I am working with too, of learning how to eat properly."

Building Networks

Perhaps the advocates' most unique contribution is the establishment of a network among agencies within and outside the community. Establishing these organizational links provides opportunities for health promotion at a variety of different sites. One advocate explained: "You learn from other people. By networking we learn about other organizations and then they connect us with other things and then we get training from them also." The advocates work hard to maintain these contacts, and these efforts in turn keep a positive image of what they contribute to the host agency. One advocate observed: "You want to leave a good impression, because you want to always, always want to go back . . . and they always will, you know, have opened arms for you." Another advocate points out the importance of a good local reputation: "They would say, 'OK, so-and-so knows that you did this over there . . . And it was great.' So that is how a lot of our contacts are . . . sometimes it is by word of mouth, not our business cards."

These contacts are also used to help individual clients solve their problems. One advocate explained: "There is all these agencies and organizations that provide so much information, support. And people that live around there, they have all these services provided and they don't know of these organizations and agencies that provide these services for them."

Another advocate said:

I got a lot of resources on different drug rehab centers. . . . A lot of people run out of food, you know, the end of the month. . . . I know different places I can send some for that, and clothes. . . . They don't understand when they're on public aid that public aid will help them out . . . and that way the kids and them don't have to suffer with sleeping on the floor.

By integrating their ties with organizations and their knowledge of life in the community, advocates are able to act as liaisons between community residents and agencies. Because advocates understand the clients' situations so well, they are able to plead the client's cause effectively with external agencies. For example, the advocate can help a social worker understand why a particular client might not have kept an appointment:

The caseworker sends you a letter and some of the apartments . . . they don't have mail box doors on there . . . sometimes it be kids . . .

tear it up. . . . So if you never receive it, you know nothing about your appointment. . . . They might get a letter on the 20th saying come to public aid office and sometimes they don't have carfare and sometime they don't have a phone, so they have [no] other choice, if they can't borrow no money, they miss that appointment hoping that next month they can get their check and reschedule.

The Challenges of the Job

The advocates all agree that their job demands a high degree of autonomy, self-determination and an open-ended commitment. Advocates serve clients, and thus orient their efforts to client and community needs rather than the needs of an employer. While a conventional job comes complete with a list of tasks to be completed, advocates create their own goals and activities. For most of the advocates these conditions were a positive feature of the job. "This job that I do now, I mean it is so interesting and it's unique, you know? It's different. God, it's not the same thing all the time, you know? It changes. You do a little bit of everything." Another advocate enthused:

> To me, every day I look forward to coming here, like going to different meetings, I meet people, going, like "specially when I go to the Unity House, I run into a lot of people who might not have food . . . and they used to come to Unity and I be telling them different places to go to and I be telling them about public aid. They make me feel good to know this information so I can help people in my community. I wish while I was on public aid, that people, you know, told me different things."

Being an advocate not only presents challenges in terms of responsibility and scope, it also is a physically active job, which many advocates really enjoyed. As one advocate observed:

> I worked before and it could be overbearing. They don't give you time to breathe. But this program you get to see a lot of outside and what is going on in the community. Before, you was like just going to a space and you were there from 8:45 A.M.–3:45 P.M. See? You never get to see the outside. You hear what I am saying? But with this particular job, you get to see how things really go. You really can get to be there. Or even to participate sometimes, or even go under cover sometimes to find good things.

However, the open-ended nature of their job was also sometimes stressful. One advocate recalled:

> It is frustrating when you have to go make the contacts. But don't get me wrong. I will do them. But it's frustrating, you know . . . from day to day you've got to really set your files and go back through your

contacts, and now what is this agency going to need this time from me? It's not like they are going to be calling. You have to in turn get on the phone and do some calling. You just can't sit there, OK? At first, I could not stand it. I said "There is no way." But then after it started to rolling, you done . . . say you did your FALP [First Aid for Little People] over here for this agency maybe two or three times. And then you went down to Red Cross and you did CPR. You was over here and you did parenting. And you was here and you done made all these rounds. Now where? There's a lot out there to do but you've got to find it, you see, yourself. And if it was just another way, it would be swell. But you must find it, and it's there. It could be very frustrating. That one can really . . . tire you out.

The advocate role requires relatively high levels of oral and written communication skills for workers who may only have a high school education, which was especially hard for those for whom English was unfamiliar. One advocate said: "Only times I am very frustrated is when I have to speak in front of a lot of people in English. That's the only thing. Or when I can have my idea complete in English and people say, 'Do you want to say this?'" Because their work is complex, documenting their activities on a brief form was also frustrating, especially for advocates with limited English. As one advocate complained:

I don't like to do encounter forms. . . . First of all because my handwriting and my spelling is not correct, not so good. . . . Then, I don't know if I can explain . . . a big problem, for words, it's hard for me. Another one is because they don't teach exactly what does it mean. Each thing. And I am confused about them. Another one is because sometimes we saw them, the clients, two or three times, and I don't see the necessity to fill it out one or two times. . . . One client, she told me that she talked to someone because she wants an abortion. And when she explained to me, I said what am I going to say in my encounter forms. I have to write down . . . what was their problem . . . I can't explain everything that she told me. Maybe just financial problems and that's it. But it was more than a financial problem. Psychological and things like that.

Another set of frustrations the advocates experienced related to the relatively low level of reward and limited opportunity for advancement they experienced. "I think that the work that an advocate does . . . I think there should be more money. That disappoints me. I think we should be getting paid more money." Another commented: "That's the biggest issue. Fine, you have benefits and this and that. But you can't eat off your benefits." Unlike many other low-paying jobs, after-hours work did not receive special compensation. "They don't pay you overtime. It's just [compensation] time. So say I was at a meeting for two hours, plus transportation, three hours. That's what, 20 something dollars. And then I have to pay the baby-sitter."

Evaluating Success as an Advocate

The advocates discussed at length how they evaluated their performance, and the intensity of these exchanges clearly revealed how engaged they all were in their work. The advocates agreed that the most gratifying part of being an advocate was being able to see positive evidence of their accomplishments. Some advocates pointed to clients' continued use of their services and their referrals to others as a sign that their work was effective.

> If they don't see results, they don't come back. It's because we, especially myself, try to be very understandable and. . . . "I'm going to really try to help you. Even though I can't have everything in my hands now, I really want to help you. And I'm going to do it." And that's when the people come back.

Another observed: "They go there to see and then we come back with more people, you know, with families, with friends they send over." Others point to concrete accomplishments with clients as evidence of success. One advocate recalled her success in a case of child abuse: "I gave her some pamphlets on [child abuse]. And she had told me, 'Well, I stopped my friend from beating the children. I told my friend don't whip the children anymore.'" Another advocate recalled with satisfaction helping a new immigrant negotiate the system: "He is about fifteen years old and he is new to the United States . . . he has been here a year and he wanted to go to high school. But he didn't know what to do or how to go about it. And I was able to help him."

For some advocates, the determination of their clients is another source of satisfaction with the job they do. One advocate recalled a particular client who affected her greatly:

> Life was falling apart, this girl didn't have no food, no rent, no money, no day care. . . . But the thing is, she gave me so much inspiration because she would call me every day and ask me, 'Do you think you could get me into school?' I didn't know how to do it and it was my first client. But I did call some people. I got on the phone and I called and called. And then when we finally got her in school, we found her a day care program.

Another advocate summed it up: "In the community there don't exist another project like this. OK, it is complete. They really help people to do for themselves."

Just as the advocates take great pride in their positive accomplishments, they also feel personal hurt and disappointment when clients do not follow through or fall back into negative behaviors.

> Here I am giving my time to this one particular client, you know, I set up appointments, I make phone calls, I give up my time to help them out with a problem that they have and then . . . after all that, they just

sit at home or they're not interested in doing nothing else about it, when I could have taken the time that I spent with this one particular client, I could have spent it with another one that was really in need. Or I could have spent it doing something else.

Another advocate echoed the same sentiments: "That's when you sort of like lose trust . . . trust in a particular client."

Being an Advocate

With this job, you get in touch with human beings. You deal with humans. You become human. You become more human yourself, because you are not even thinking about the paycheck anymore, you are not thinking about, you know. . . . "It is time for me to go home now." Because sometimes at the last minute, you might get a phone call and it might be a family and they don't have anything to eat and you just. . . . You're on your way home, but there is just no way that you can say "No." You turn back and go back in and try to find them something.

The Advocate and the Work Team

The advocates identified three important aspects of their relationships: teamwork, friction, and friendship. Teamwork was important because it made the advocates more effective. For some advocates, this was the first time they really experienced the benefits of teamwork. One advocate observed:

I remember thinking of myself, "Oh, gee, I like working by myself," you know? . . . But in this situation I think I am . . . changing my mind on that, because you learn a lot of them have had more experience than I have. So they know things. And they are very good about giving help, you know.

The team provided support and encouragement. More experienced team members served as role models and mentors for new advocates.

When I started, it was a challenge for me to work with people who have very different ideas. And then we have to put all our ideas together to get something. And I was very quiet because I always apologize about my English. And they really helped me a lot, you know. They didn't criticize me, you know, about my English. And they teach me about the community, where to go, how to prepare presentations, health presentations, how to talk to the people.

Advocates also mentioned that they felt safer in the neighborhood working in a team: "Mercy, it is not safe to work nowhere now by yourself. . . . If something happens . . . the other advocate can always be there to help. It is good to go in pairs now."

There was also occasional friction and negative experiences related to the team. The most serious challenges to team cohesion occurred on the rare occasions when one advocate hurt another in some way. One advocate discussed her sense of betrayal when some money was taken by another advocate:

> When my wallet came up out of the purse at the site . . . that was the first time . . . it happened at the site, you see. And I was fortunate enough to get it back. And that made me want to not be there any more. That made me feel very uncomfortable because you don't know what the person is going to do next, you see? Because you don't think of a person like that, you always think nice. . . . I mean, you have been nice and you would think of a person as you would yourself.

Although an apology was given and the money returned, the advocate felt that her relationship with that person could never be the same. Other advocates mentioned occasional friction of the sort to be expected when many people work together in a small space: "Sometimes I try to stay at a distance because we all are different. Different personalities. And then sometimes attitudes arise. Sometimes I feel as though one of my coworkers don't want [me] to be around. I just stay to myself." Another source of friction was occasional feelings that one person was not pulling their weight or not as committed: "She works her tail off and the other one just sits around and loafs around . . . and I'm tired of seeing it." One advocate complained that sometimes others were not interested in hearing about her experiences or in sharing their resources:

> I might come in and say, "Well, girls, guess what I encountered today?" And you know, they don't want to listen to me now. So, I keep it to myself. So I might ask, "Do you know of any resources where I could tell one of my clients?" For instance, someone might need a bed, and they probably don't want to share with me and mine. So I just try to find it out on my own.

Despite the problems advocates sometimes encountered in maintaining a cohesive team, they also found that working together developed deeply meaningful relationships: "I was able to share with them some things that I would not have shared with, let's say a family member. . . . No matter how we bicker . . . and get on each other's nerves . . . there is something there. . . . We share a lot." Perhaps the most eloquent description of this relationship came from one advocate, who said:

> You know what, I feel like the advocates are lovely. For one thing, everybody's got a heart. I mean we work and we feel. We feel what is going on out there and . . . I have worked with other people, and it

was not that they didn't have feelings or that they didn't have a heart, but they didn't show it. And then we might be frustrated . . . but all in all I know we go home with a good feeling. And so I am close to them, you know? We are different persons, so we don't see everything as a whole; we have got differences in opinions. But we do care for the people, and that is what we are there for.

Relations with Nurses

Advocates see their nurse as their team leader, mentor, supporter, and resident expert. The nurse's special health knowledge and experience is a critical and unique contribution which the entire team relies upon. One advocate described the role of the nurse this way: "We are the community people. We know how to talk to the people, but when it comes down to a matter of health, that is you know, an emergency or something, then she has to come in." Another observed:

It is beautiful to have a nurse. Because we run into things, since we are not a medical terminology person. So it is so good and I hope they always will keep a nurse behind the advocates. Things that we can't relate to, like little rashes. We might tell them they got herpes or something! We can identify it and make them feel good right then and there. I learn to do [blood] pressures just by having a nurse there. And so I was so glad to know that they had a nurse. She has got a lot of knowledge on things, and that helps the program a whole lot.

As one advocate described: "She will go with us and do some of our workshops, you know? She works with us. Then she'll sit in to see how we perform . . . yes, she is very supportive." Another advocate: "If I wanted to do a presentation . . . I might ask her certain questions about, like 'How exactly do drugs affect the body?' . . . And she knows a lot about these types of things. And that helps a lot." The nurse also provides more personal support and advice: "She always is there. You know, if we need to call her in the middle of the night, she's there. And she's very interested in us."

The advocates find the nurse to be more flexible than a boss in a conventional job: "To me that's the best boss that you can ever have. 'Cause like you know, you have a problem, you sit down, and she talks to you, she understands. Like some bosses are real, real quick on you. She's not like that. She's not looking over your shoulder like some bosses." At the same time, the nurse sets high standards for the quantity and quality of work as well as for the commitment, creativity, and energy advocates should bring to their job. One advocate described the process: "She will warn you first, this and that, you know. 'You are crooking up, okay?' And then you know to straighten it up because she knows that you got good intentions in you. And when you don't, you can make it very hot for yourself."

The relationship between the advocate and nurse is very close and personal. Not surprisingly, one team of advocates was very stressed when they experienced a change in their nurse. One person eventually left the job, and blamed some of her dissatisfaction on the new nurse: "The whole team fell apart when the nurse left . . . and to me it has never gotten back up again. . . . The new nurse came in at a bad time . . . and it's been downhill ever since." Another advocate on the same team adapted and came to appreciate the unique capacities of each nurse:

> The first nurse that I had was very sensitive to community and very sensitive to the different cultures, and I guess because she was traveling a lot. And her personality was very kind, very sweet, you know. And we can be very friendly . . . easy . . . very well friends. She really tries to trust people. In working with the new one, in the beginning it was very hard because she didn't have too much sensitivity to different cultures . . . she's really learned fast. And also she's very strong. She's very strict. And that's what I like of her. . . . She really wants to have done something before the project is gone.

The advocates have a strong appreciation of the nurse and her contributions to the project:

> Matter of fact, somebody told me that I put my boss on a pedestal. But I feel . . . first of all to admire because she does so much. She would be everywhere, places where I would not go. She goes to the little families in the ghettos and these people actually like her. I mean they won't welcome me, but they will say, 'OK, come in.' You know? I will sit outside and wait for her. Sometimes I will be so scared to go into these places. But, yeah, I look up to her because she is doing a lot. And she is doing it. From the bottom of her heart, this is what she likes to do.

Relations with University Staff

The university staff is a much more diverse group with more varied tasks and levels of involvement with the advocates. Contacts between the advocates and the university staff were not as frequent or as intense as their relationships within the nurse/advocate team. The advocates talked about these relationships less and their feelings about them were not nearly as intense, but they recognized that the university staff brought ideas, knowledge, connections, and material resources to the project which enabled the project to function:

> I think that we need the university . . . being out here [at the university] has been more helpful than working from an agency that was just out there . . . because you guys are here and the people that are out

there are used to everything that's going on out there. And those agencies they have in the storefront, everything is day to day.

Another advocate observed: "I guess it's because you're able to take it back to other people. I know that, like let's say [a university staff person], she writes up these grants and is able to get jobs . . . and train people that are able to go out there and help and develop." One advocate praised the staff for always trying to find out what the advocates needed: "They say, 'Well . . . we are short of moneys. We'll see what we can do.' And to me that is better than, 'No, no. I don't see no way.'"

The advocates also appreciated the respect and support the university staff gave them for their activities. One advocate commented:

OK, maybe the people that have like more education than you, higher education. Right. Just knowing that when we come back and we inform them of our opinions, our ideas, our experience from being out in our community, what's going on, what we have done and it's like, "Wow!" They see it to be as a wonderful thing, a great thing that we're doing.

The staff meetings were the most frequent format in which the advocates interacted regularly with the university staff in their roles as project leaders. Some of the advocates liked these meetings and valued their ability to participate: "Being in a staff meeting with the heavy shots . . . that's what I call you . . . it makes me feel good. It makes me feel good to be part of that team. I am learning. I am sitting in. I put out and then I soak a lot in." Some advocates complained that the ideas of the staff were often too abstract for them to readily understand or use in the community: "Really when they had the staff meetings, the stuff they was talking about, I didn't know nothing about and a lot of my coworkers feel that way. The stuff you talk about, we be lost. We don't understand." Another commented: "When I come up here and we have those staff meetings, I find them to be useful, because I learn new things, information that comes then, you know, like what's going on." A few discussed how they found the meetings difficult at first and gradually learned to appreciate them over time. One advocate observed that at first she had been quiet: "But I found out that if we are doing something in the community, you know, it is good to let them know." They also found that they gradually gained the self-confidence to participate more freely in the meetings.

Some felt that the university staff took the credit for the advocate's hard work. As project leaders, the university staff made scholarly presentations and wrote publications and pamphlets, but as one advocate put it: "A lot of the people here, they don't know what's really going on because they're hardly ever out there." One advocate was especially critical:

Well at first I was, 'Wow, I'm going to be working at the university!' But after a year, two years, and I started hearing the advocates from other sites talking and I started to realize we were doing the dirty work for these people. You know? I feel like they just put us out there to do the dirty work. They're getting all the credit. You know, they are showing their statistics and their videotapes [about the work of the advocate and multidisciplinary teams] all over the country, all over the world. They get the credit, not us.

This feeling was exacerbated by the advocates' awareness that university staff had much higher salaries and more privileged lives than they did. Personal relationships with the university staff also varied. Several advocates commented on the close relationships they had developed with university staff: "I guess because . . . after the training. . . . I worked at the university. . . . So I got along with them real fine, better because I was up there every day." Other advocates, however, did not share this feeling: "Working with the university staff . . . sometimes I don't understand a lot of them, OK. I feel as though, like they feel a little superior to us. It is not a close relationship, as it should be."

How Advocates See Their Community

Advocates perceive their communities as having serious and pervasive problems, but also as having resources that can help to solve these difficulties. When asked what the community's most serious problems were, two-thirds of the advocates named drugs, gangs, and gang-related violence: "The drugs are something that as long as there's poverty, they're never going to get rid of them, the drugs and the gangs. They just move on. If you push it from here, it just moves on to the other corner. In our area, the police are just as involved in it as the kids are." These problems lead to isolation, fear, and environmental degradation. One advocate saw community involvement as a function of these factors:

> With the gangs and the drugs there's a lot of people afraid to come out. Like they might come out I say once—they take the kids to school, like go to Jewel's [a local supermarket] or whatever and go pick their kids up from school. After school, they's stuck in the house and I believe that's why a lot of people's don't attend these meetings because they are afraid to come out, if it ain't drug dealers that's approaching them, it's the gangs.

Drug use, and the lack of available treatment programs, were also linked to homelessness. Lack of education, and its impact on the ability to get good jobs, was the second most frequently discussed problem.

> [In the advocate's community] I would say that we are not well educated. We are not. Most of us are Spanish or blacks and we are not well educated, for whatever the reasons. Some of us have kids too early, or

came from another country. It is a lot of struggle, so these people
don't finish school. They don't have the motivation to go back to
school.

The lack of jobs and unemployment as well as lack of safe housing and homelessness were also mentioned frequently. Immigrants' difficulties in language,
communication, accessing jobs, healthcare, and information and general
adjustment were also important priorities for those advocates working in the
Latino community: "There is a lot of immigrants in that area, people who have
just come here, and they have tough times because of the language problems.
And getting things like public aid and stuff like that. So that is another big
problem . . . having access to the system."

Problems within families were also mentioned frequently. Teen pregnancy
and the lack of good child care and parenting were also seen as important community problems.

There's not enough guidance at a young age. There's a lot of single
parents. A lot of women have just one thing on their mind, getting
their public aid check, which they get once a month. They go out
there . . . and a lot of them don't even bother with . . . spending any
time with their kids. A lot of young, single parents. Then the father,
you don't know where he is at. A lot of fathers don't care once they
separate from the mother.

Another described how adolescent pregnancy was a more serious obstacle
today since many grandmothers are unwilling or unable to care for the baby:
"How can they go back to school if they don't have nobody to keep that baby
for them?" The advocates also see domestic violence as both serious and difficult to change: "I mean you can only do so much. . . . You try to get them help
and you go so far and then they just reject everything you've done for them.
You feel frustrated."

Advocates pointed out the multiple links between health and socioeconomic problems: "If you are not working, how can you get the proper things
to keep yourself like fed properly, and keep yourself warm?" Another advocate
observed:

Since these people are low income, most of them . . . they face a lot of
nutrition problems, either because they don't have the money or they
don't have the food or the knowledge to fix the right kinds of meals.
So they are always sick. Some of them are overweight or too slim. So
they have got a lot of health issues.

Advocates feel that to address these maladies, basic social and economic
resources need to be enhanced in the community: "Give minorities more jobs.
Give them the opportunities to work, make some work. I don't think it is

because they just don't want to. It is not nothing available for them." Another advocate points out that not just any job will do: "Because . . . you talk to a drug dealer and . . . find him a job making $5 or $6 an hour . . . that's gonna sound like peanuts to him, because he's used to making a thousand dollars, two thousand dollars . . . a day."

Local solutions depend upon the community leaders who are already working for improvements and some sense of social justice:

> I know quite a few peoples that in the community who concerned about drugs and gangs. For instance, they see drug dealers out in the corner, they do call the police. There's about three people [on] my floor who use drugs and would love to have drugs sold in their apartment. They know a couple of us ain't gonna stand for that, so they don't do it on our floor.

Advocates see themselves and community-based primary health care as only part of the solution for their communities. However, the advocates are optimistic that over time they can make a difference. One woman summed it up:

> I think that we can do a lot. Because in my neighborhood, when I first got into the training, people . . . you know, they didn't know what I was doing . . . but . . . about a month ago this girl came in about 1 A.M. at night knocking on my door, to tell me she was homeless. So it's around my block—everybody knows and everybody's proud of me. They look at me in a different light. I feel like they feel like I am doing something for them . . . yes, we can change the world. If we can get them to work with us and teach them what we know, and change.

How Advocates See the University

The advocates discussed the mixed feelings both they and members of their community have about the role of the university in promoting community health. Advocates appreciated both the resources and the reputation of the university. Association with the university brings access to a great deal of faculty expertise, physical resources such as rooms for meetings, and advantages such as employee benefits: "Since the university is a big institution, they can serve people there. We can have access to many things. Like cultural things, like health, like use these services like libraries. For example, for the project, they have our office here. You know, more space." Some advocates found that being associated with the university helped to open doors to them: "When we call and we say we're from the University of Illinois and the College of Nursing . . . people look at you like they know what you're talking about." However, recognition of the university in the community is not always positive:

> Most people when they think of the university they think of research. It's not a safe place. . . . Right now some of the . . . parents think of

the university as they come into school as sort of research. They may not be doing that, but that's what they look at. What does the university really do?

Another advocate always introduces herself without mentioning the university because if you mention the university: ". . . they feel as though that you are working for a bunch of white people."

A major issue for many community residents is the lack of long-term commitment. Advocates report that community residents ask: "'Why did you come in here with this and have us all charged up . . . and then tomorrow it's gone?' Even if they are told that this is only for this amount of time or whatever, they figure 'Why can't we have this to stay here?'" Another issue is accessibility: "Going to their community . . . you will get a better turnout than inviting somebody to come down to the university, because you don't know if they have the carfare." One advocate summed up the mixed community reactions to the university when she said:

> For some people in the community, it is like a threat, like well, why should they be interested in us. Or the people who live over here in the neighborhood of the university, they feel that they lost by the university . . . then we try to tell them, "Hey listen, look what they are giving you back." But then again, some of the places you go in you say "University of Illinois" and they open the doors wide open. So you walk right in. . . . So sometimes you are welcome, sometimes you are not welcome. But as far as personal, I feel good, and I feel like I am there doing a job and the university's letting me be able to go out there and talk to these people.

Another advocate pointed out: "That's where the advocates come in and they have to play defense for the university to reassure these people that 'No, they're here to help. They're not here to take advantage of you or find out what your health problems are and run with it or things of that nature.'" Thus, the advocates can promote university involvement in the community both by introducing university projects and vouching for the university's intentions.

How Advocates See the Healthcare System

The advocates had mainly negative perceptions of the healthcare system and found it inadequate to meet their community's health needs. Their first complaint was the lack of quality services in their community:

> The doctors are . . . you know, they are not putting too much in the neighborhood. I mean, we have got the [local] clinic and we have got some medical centers. Those are good if you can get in. But the demand is so heavy that if a parent goes there with their child and you

know, you are going to sit there all day long, you are going to go home and give him an aspirin. You know, and wait until it gets worse.

Another added: "... or the health services might be around, but people can't afford it. Because of, you know, just the high pricing of first visit to a doctor, thirty, forty bucks. I mean, Wow! That's too much!"

Another serious complaint about the health system related to cultural and language barriers between healthcare providers and community residents. In explaining why it was important to have a nurse on the team, one advocate highlighted some of the barriers that keep people from getting adequate care:

> We had a lady, she was a victim of domestic violence. I said, "Listen, you know, this lady is here, she is running a fever, she doesn't have medical benefits, no medical card, no money, and I don't know what to do with her, but I can't tell her to go home, because you know, I don't know what is going on." When the nurse came and she said, "Listen, this is really serious," she found a doctor who would see her. As an advocate probably I would not have got her that far. I would have tried, but I couldn't have. But she knew the right medical words to say, from a medical point of view, which I didn't know.

Effects on Personal Lives

All of the advocates described their experiences as life changing. Their relationships with their families changed as they incorporated what they had learned into their own lives. Learning to balance the demands of their work and their personal lives was a major issue. The advocates also discussed the knowledge, skills, and self-awareness they had gained. Finally, the advocates observed how their perspectives about themselves and their plans for the future had changed over time.

Relationships with Family. Most advocates were able to share their knowledge and understanding with their families. One advocate discussed how being an advocate enabled her to discuss serious issues with her adolescent children: "For myself, I've been able to use it for talking to my kids. . . . And then too, like for my daughters, my older daughters, I talk to them about AIDS. I talk to them about STDs and I've been able to talk free with them about a lot of stuff." However, sometimes advocates found that the things they could do to help clients they weren't able to do with their own families. Family problems sometimes interfered with their ability to work. This was especially difficult when women were experiencing problems in their own family similar to the problems they were addressing with clients or through teaching:

> We help so many people and yet sometimes I feel that if something happened to me at the house, that I've been real upset, I don't think

that I could sit there and give advice to somebody. No. You can't do this and this and that, because your mind is not clear. Okay, how could you go into a support group and run a parental stress group, a support group for women, if you're the person who comes in all stressed out?

Balancing Work and Personal Lives. All women who work and have family obligations face the challenge of too little time and the need to balance their time and energies. There were several factors that made this especially difficult for the advocates. The high level of commitment required to be a health advocate placed unusually heavy demands on the advocates' time and energies for a relatively low-level job. Advocates often found themselves working beyond the end of their paid day to help clients, and also had difficulty drawing the line between work and nonwork because their neighbors asked for help outside work hours: "Is it a nuisance to get calls? Sometimes. It's like, 'Come on, I work Monday through Friday. I want the weekend off.' But I don't mind. I guess with this type of job, being a health advocate is a 24-hour on-call job." Evening meetings were a common occurrence and a source of additional strain. One advocate who was leaving the program felt that the evening meetings were too much for her, especially as a single mother:

> We're expected to. We're not forced to work, we're expected to. They leave it up to us. But they're not going to catch me at no meeting at 7 or 8 or 9 or 10 o'clock at night. I'm sorry. It's not worth that. It's because of my family, number one. Because, as somebody put it in the office where I work, "My family comes first." I said, "Well, mine does too." And I'm not going to be running around in the middle of the night without transportation, waiting for a bus. I said, "I'm sorry, I'm not going to risk my life for $6.00 an hour."

On the other hand, advocates appreciated the more flexible nature of their jobs because it made meeting family responsibilities easier. One mother said: "That is the one part of my job that I think I would say that I like the most. You know, flexible, that when my kids are sick or whatever I can take off." Even if the advocates were not working, they found themselves worrying about the job and their clients:

> You know, sometimes it's hard to leave your job at work. Honestly, I have found myself, I am at home and I could be looking at TV or just reading and all of a sudden like, something that happened that day or that week pops in my mind. And I start thinking about it. I start wondering, "Oh, I wonder how she's doing?"

Working as an advocate often meant that the advocates no longer had much leisure time to be with their family and friends. Moreover, their families and neighbors were unfamiliar with the idea of a demanding job so they were not very tolerant of the advocates' job demands. As one advocate described her friends' reactions: "Well, they don't get to see much of me. 'Since you started to work, we hardly ever hear from you. How are you?' You know, this kind of thing. . . . And I really don't get to visit as much." Over time, the advocates gradually developed strategies for balancing their lives and setting limits on their availability. One single mother captured the realities for many when she explained:

> I really try not to let work get to me. Sometimes I get off work and I be tired and I got a six-year-old daughter. When I come into the house, she be telling me she needs help with her homework and she says, "I don't know how to do this." Some days when I come home, I'm not just for it and then I be a little mad and then I say let me just get myself together and then I go on and help her. But sometimes, you know, I wish I didn't have no kids. That way you come home and you can just go to bed or whatever. And sometimes when I come home, the phone is ringing and somebody wants their blood pressure taken and sometimes I just don't be in the mood for it, but I go on and do it. I don't want to turn my back on them.

Change and Self-Discovery. The advocates gained knowledge, cognitive and interpersonal skills, as well as self-confidence as a result of their many learning experiences, continuing education, and work: "It improves your reading skills. This program would improve your writing skills. . . . Working with this program, you will learn to think. You will learn to jot down things. You will learn to update things." Another advocate described how she had gained valuable skills in self-presentation and confidence in herself, as well as health knowledge:

> First of all . . . we learn about ourselves, our body and everything. Second one, I don't have to be more afraid to talk in public. Especially in Spanish, I am not afraid. Something I can say. I can understand more about different things, you know, different topics. I can go and talk to the senator and I can be comfortable to talk to him.

One advocate described how she had learned to be assertive when meeting resistance: "I believe there is something else you can do to help me here. And it is no more taking 'No' for an answer until it is just wiped off, taken out of the book, and up in Italy some place. So you don't take no for an answer, no more, because I know better now." Another advocate summed up what she had gained:

> Because of my experience that I've learned. And I don't need a bachelor's or a master's. It's there, I've learned it. Everything that I learned

dealing with the people. Other . . . people have to go to school and get a bachelor's and I don't need that. I just learned it and I know it. And I know how to deal with people and I know how to do this, and I know how to do that. And I learned it all from here. So thanks to the university (laughs).

Advocates had the opportunity to work with others with a variety of educational backgrounds and jobs. This exposure also greatly increased the advocates' desire for more learning:

> Before coming into this program, I said, "Oh, I am not going to go back to school. I am just going to find me a job and call it a shot." And this program makes you want to go back to school and get all kinds of bachelor degrees. Just want to reach out and help people much more than you could ever in your lifetime. That is what it does for me; it made me feel good about myself. . . . People have misjudged me in a lot of ways. My self-esteem in getting before people to express myself. . . . I wouldn't dare. But being in a program like this one, you learn to stand tall and learn to look out and say what you have to say. And there it is. I have come a long way.

In fact, many of the advocates accomplished these goals and moved on to more advanced positions, nearly all in the helping professions. It was difficult for some to balance their newfound aspirations with their current life circumstances and educational record, so that they had to accept that certain options were not presently realistic for them. As one advocate observed: "If this training would have been here like, let's say, ten years ago, I probably would have been a nurse right now. Yeah, I would have gotten more involved. Even though they say it's never too late, but I don't know. . . . I'm still thinking about it." Often, the advocates were able to find a compromise between their dreams and realities.

The advocates' experiences had built their overall self-esteem and confidence as well as specific capacities. Through repeated success in public speaking and leading groups, advocates built both self-confidence and positive self-images. Their growing self-esteem led advocates to change their views of themselves and their future, to "dream bigger dreams":

> If I was still at home, and I would have never taken this job or this training, I would not think like this. I would still be thinking ten years behind what I'm thinking now, ten years ahead. So it has because of what I've seen and what I've learned and the people that I've dealt with. I have gotten more perspective on it right now. I can appreciate what I have because I've seen people who don't have nothing. And I appreciate more what I have, because compared to what those people that I deal with, you know, it was depressing. So I think that I have appreciated life more now.

DISCUSSION

It is important to compare the way advocates view their role with the views of health professionals and university staff. The advocates share many perspectives: In particular, they clearly see their role as a bridge between the community and the wider world. They describe how many of the stresses of their job originate in this effort to bridge the gap between two different worlds. Moreover, in their own lives many of them struggle with the issue of how far beyond the community they want and are able to go. The advocates remain rooted at the individual and family level in their perspectives, rarely concerning themselves with overall program outcomes. Instead they evaluate success by what their work does for their neighbors and their immediate community. The advocates viewed their sphere of work also from a very local perspective, being most involved in their immediate work team of nurse-leader and fellow advocates. While they identified strongly with their communities, they retained deep ambivalence toward both the university and the community.

The advocates clearly saw unique elements in the way they were able to promote health compared to a professional. The lived experiences they bring from the community, the health knowledge they bring to the community, and the network of connections to agencies and organizations they create in the community all enable them to serve as effective role models, teachers, and change agents. This insiders' view of their role is parallel to the conceptual model of their position as a bridge between the community and the healthcare system/university discussed by program developers in other chapters. This congruence between advocates and professionals in the understanding of the advocate role is an important validation of our conceptual model.

One theme running through the advocates' discussions was the persistent issue of boundaries. The role of the health advocate (unlike their previous work experience) was highly fluid. The job itself required many after-hours work, especially attendance at community and group meetings in the evening. The job also demanded a commitment to the issues and individuals served that made it hard to just walk away at the end of the day. Thinking about the job, personal issues, future plans, distress of clients, and other concerns spilled over into "non-work" time. At the same time, the job itself offered greater flexibility in time use, because advocates were given compensatory time off for their evening activities rather than overtime. This made it possible for advocates to integrate various personal and family obligations into their working day. Few descriptions are available about how working class women integrate their multiple responsibilities. While their challenges are in many ways similar to more affluent working women, their lack of resources and their presence in a milieu that does not value career involvement make meeting these challenges more stressful.

One of the most striking elements of the advocates' story is the degree to which they experienced personal growth. They developed commitment to working, future education, and a career. They developed a more positive sense of themselves and an impressive set of capacities for change and reflection.

Being an advocate expanded their horizons and deepened their commitment to helping others. In light of current efforts to end welfare, the capacities of these women to grow when provided a supportive and engaging work opportunity are inspiring. Developers of community-based primary health care demonstration projects often expect conventional community and individual health outcomes for those served to provide indicators of program success. However, the development of leadership capacities among the local residents who work as health advocates is an equally important contribution. The changes in the health advocates will continue to enrich their lives and make contributions to their community well beyond the life of a demonstration project.

Chapter 5

A Nurse/Health Advocate Team to Empower Hispanic Immigrant Women

KAREN A. BUCK
PATRICIA FOX

A special thanks must go to Ms. Martha Prado-Gonzáles, community health advocate, for her assistance with the interviews. Her help was invaluable, and working with her taught me many things about community empowerment. Also, thanks to Dr. Beverly J. McElmurry for her encouragement, probing questions, and interest in this project and to Dr. Chang Park who helped formulate ideas in the early stages of this project. Finally, we would like to acknowledge Maria Vasquez and Nina Buck for their work in translating and transcribing the interviews. Soli Deo gloria.

INTRODUCTION

As the state with the fifth largest Hispanic population (Mattson, 1990), Illinois has funded a program to improve the health status of its Hispanic immigrants. In 1991, the Primary Health Care in Urban Communities (PHCUC) project was awarded funds under a subcontract from the Chicago Department of Public Health's Hispanic Coalition to assist in the implementation of the State Legalization Impact Assistance Grant (SLIAG). The PHCUC uses a primary health care (PHC) approach to improve the health of underserved communities, through the work of a nurse and community health advocate (CHA) "who collaborate in defining, developing, and implementing strategies responsive to the concerns and essential health needs of community residents" (McElmurry et al., 1990, p. 122). The target communities for the SLIAG project were Humboldt Park, West Town, Avondale, and Hermosa on the west side of Chicago.

At the time this study was conducted, a registered nurse worked part-time with the CHA. The CHA is a member of the community who has received training in health promotion, and she functions as an agent of change in the community with the goal of mobilizing community members to improve their health (Swider & McElmurry, 1990). This is accomplished by a variety of means including: health fairs, parenting classes, assistance with transportation, health education, translation, helping with public assistance applications, and finding clothing and food. Underlying all of these services is the social support that the CHA provides to those she is in contact with. Individuals and families are referred to the CHA, and she works with them to help resolve their problems.

This nurse/health advocate team worked to improve the health of the communities it serves. Through their involvement with individuals and families in the community, the team has sought to make health and healthcare more attainable for the community as a whole.

Other studies have examined various components of the SLIAG community health advocacy team. Keeney (1993), used quantitative and qualitative methods to describe the perceived barriers to healthcare services among Hispanic immigrants in the community served by the nurse/health advocate team. Another study investigated the efficacy of the community health advocacy team by looking at completion rate of referrals and the factors that were associated with successful follow through on referrals (Barron, 1994).

"[A] goal of the PHCUC is the empowerment of community members in areas related to health" (Swider & McElmurry, 1990, p. 14). The purpose of this study was to elicit testimony from Hispanic immigrant women regarding their interaction with a nurse/health advocate team. It was designed to ascertain if their experience with the team reflected empowerment. This purpose was achieved through conducting a series of interviews with participants in the SLIAG program.

EMPOWERMENT

Gibson (1991) defines empowerment as "a social process of recognizing, promoting, and enhancing people's abilities to meet their own needs, solve their own problems, and mobilize the necessary resources in order to feel in control of their own lives. . . . [it is] a process of helping people assert control over the factors which affect their health" (p. 359). In an extensive literature review of empowerment and community participation, Walls (1996) describes seven aspects of empowerment that have emerged from the literature. These include relationship, experience, self-knowledge, trust, action, valuing of derived aspects (of empowerment), and caring (see Table 1 for attributes). From these aspects of empowerment, the concept of affirmative relationships emerges as the overarching principle that ties all of the various aspects of empowerment together. Walls notes that these relational aspects require that each person involved in the relationship acknowledge their responsibility to contribute to the process. As Walls articulated:

> Affirmative relationships commit persons to each other through activities such as partnerships, mentoring, sharing, and/or dialogue. Aspects of empowerment such as caring, trust, and increased knowledge development also may require relationships with others. Relationship implies an ongoing process, a time needed for trust for knowledge to develop. Increases in self-knowledge, experience, and action are listed as other aspects of empowerment (p. 23).

Eng, Salmon, and Mullen (1992) outlined a theoretical framework and model for the application of empowerment to PHC. Through empowerment, "health professionals create conditions and opportunities for people to recognize that they can take power simultaneously as individuals and as a community" (p. 5). Building community responsibility and empowerment involves a mind-set shift for many nurses and other health professionals who consider themselves, rather than the community, as the impetus for change (Eng et al., 1992; Chalmers & Kristajanson, 1989; Connelly et al., 1993; Maglacas, 1988). In an empowerment model, health professionals work alongside the community and its members to improve health. This concept of working with the community was articulated in *Pedagogy of the Oppressed,* a pioneer work on empowerment by Paulo Friere (1970).

Community empowerment can be operationalized as community competence (Minkler, 1992). Cottrell (1976), in his work about mental health and community competence, suggests that community competence is the ability of a community, along with its constituent parts, to identify the needs and problems of the community, achieve a working consensus on goals and priorities, agree on the ways and means to implement the agreed-upon goals, and to collaborate effectively in the required actions. A competent community is able to

TABLE 1.
Attributes of Empowerment from a Literature Review
(Walls, 1996, p. 23).

1. Relationship (participation, partnership, mentoring, communion, dialogue, collaboration, sharing)
2. Experience (knowledge/maturity)
3. Self-knowledge (awareness)
4. Trust (of self and others, self-esteem empathy)
5. Action (change, motivation, creativity, realization of outcomes, joy in life, transcendence of ego, sense of moving toward wholeness)
6. Valuing of derived aspects of empowerment
7. Caring

interact effectively, that is, to construct and use structures that allow it to manage the problems of its collective life and its members to lead satisfying and productive lives (Wilson, 1976). Building social networks and social support within the community will enhance a community's ability to reach the goals of empowerment and competence (Israel, 1985).

Empowerment has been reflected in a variety of community health worker programs, both among the CHWs themselves and in the community. Community participation in a health fair (May, Mendelson, & Ferketich, 1995), a strong social support network formed among volunteer mothers in prenatal outreach program (Mahon, McFarlane, & Golden, 1991), improved self-esteem among volunteer mothers (Patton, 1995; Meister et al., 1992), volunteers organizing a community clothes bank (Patton, 1995), and CHWs mentoring women to become volunteer mothers (Clinton & Larner, 1988) are all indications of empowerment. The community health workers themselves had become empowered as evidenced by improved self-esteem (Patton, 1995; Bray & Edwards, 1994), increased investment in the community (May et al., 1995), and the development of leadership skills (Mahon et al., 1991).

HISPANIC IMMIGRANT WOMEN'S HEALTH ISSUES

Hispanic women immigrating to the United States face several stressors that affect their health. As they juggle financial, family, and community responsibilities, some women experience conflict and overload while others are able to successfully maintain a balance. These issues are not unique to Hispanic women, and are encountered by immigrant women from other cultural and ethnic backgrounds. "Immigrant women's health issues vary considerably with the time they have lived in the host country, social conditions at the time they arrived, and the reasons for leaving their home country" (Lipson, McElmurry, & LaRosa, 1995).

In the Hispanic-American family, the female serves as the primary care giver (Caudle, 1991; Reinert, 1986; Gonzales-Swafford & Gutierrez, 1983). Decisions about healthcare involve the whole family, and are usually made after consultation with the male who manages finances and transportation (Caudle, 1991). Once the woman has determined that a health problem is beyond her capability to treat, she may consult with a healthcare provider (Gonzales-Swafford & Gutierrez, 1983). This may occur at the same time or after the woman has sought help from family and friends and possibly a folk healer, or for a Mexican American, a *curandero* (Reinert, 1986). Since the female is the principal link between a family and the healthcare system, she has been a natural focal point of many health outreach activities in the Hispanic immigrant community.

Employment status can have both positive and negative effects on Hispanic immigrant women's health. On the one hand, immigrant women who work "report an increased sense of autonomy, more accomplishment, more confidence, and [they] enjoyed buying previously unaffordable items" (Wilson, 1995, p. 10). However, they may also find themselves working long hours for low pay along with poor job security and no hope for advancement (Juarbe, 1995). This may make it difficult for them to meet the responsibilities and expectations of their family roles (Wilson, 1995). Women who are undocumented and employed may find themselves controlled by their employer; they may be trapped in unhealthy, even abusive situations because their employer threatens to decrease income or reveal their immigration status if they do not comply with the employer's demands. If a woman is unable to find employment, she finds herself dependent on her partner or spouse for things such as transportation, money, and help with domestic activities (e.g., shopping). "For these women, their inability to independently fulfill the domestic role created a loss of a role and put stress on the conjugal relationship" (Wilson, 1995, p. 10). Some women may use sex to preserve financial security, personal protection, and emotional security; this leads to increased risk of pregnancy, sexually transmitted diseases, increased dependency, and lowered self-esteem (Wilson, 1995).

Accessing the healthcare system presents many difficulties to immigrant women including transportation, affordability, language barriers, and inconvenient office hours (Wilson, 1995). Juarbe (1995) examined the access issues that specifically affect Hispanic women, and she noted that they are more likely than Anglo women to be the head of their household, to be in poor health, to have a higher risk for chronic illness, and to live below the poverty line. Lack of education and language skills further limits the ability of many Hispanic women to acquire the knowledge necessary for them to access or use healthcare services (Juarbe, 1995). If a woman is an undocumented resident, she may not access healthcare for fear of being deported (Wilson, 1995) or because she does not have health insurance to cover the cost of service (Juarbe, 1995).

METHODOLOGY

This study was qualitative in design. The sample for this study was a convenience sample of five women who were open cases in the SLIAG program. Participants ranged in age from 28 to 43, and they were all first generation Mexican-American immigrants.

Although the primary investigator was capable of speaking and understanding some Spanish, she was not sufficiently fluent to conduct the interviews. For this reason, the CHA played a major role in the investigation process. The purpose of the study was explained to clients in Spanish by the CHA. The CHA also aided in obtaining consent and conducted the interview. During the interview, the CHA gave summary statements of the client's responses to the investigator, and the investigator sought clarification of responses and asked further questions of the client through the CHA.

Interviews were tape recorded with the client's permission. Once the interview was on tape, it was translated into English by a bilingual translator who was not involved with the project. The English translation of the interview was then transcribed by a typist. Demographic data were obtained from the client's record after the interview.

An open-ended questionnaire was used during the interview. The questionnaire was structured around four general areas reflecting the concepts of empowerment as outlined by Walls (Table 1). Topics addressed included: difficulties encountered when immigrating to the United States, the client's relationship with the health promoter, benefits of the SLIAG program to other family members and friends, and personal benefits from involvement in SLIAG.

The data collected in this study were categorized and analyzed based on the themes that emerged from the interviews. This was done according to the first phase of Leonard's (1989) hermeneutic phenomenology strategy by conducting a thematic analysis to identify the themes, code the themes, and then identify general categories that form the basis of the findings of the study. Color coding was done according to identified themes as recommended by Knafl and Webster (1988). These themes were not predetermined, but arose as similar ideas and topics became evident in the interview content. The themes served as a means for organizing the results of the study.

RESULTS

The themes that emerged from the interviews will be presented in this section. These themes categorize the descriptions of the five participants regarding their interaction with the CHA and the assistance they received from her. The three themes are as follows: (a) services provided by the CHA, (b) characteristics of the CHA, and (c) behavioral and affective responses of client.

Services Provided by the CHA

The participants discussed a variety of services the CHA provided for them. These services included translation, transportation, referral, and education.

Most of the women mentioned their inability to understand or speak English as one of the difficulties that they had when first immigrating to the United States. One woman described her experience on a public transportation bus:

> One of the difficulties I encountered here was when I would get on the bus and I didn't understand what the bus driver was saying and that they want the money to go in when you come in, and so they get very aggravated because you don't understand what they're saying. And so when you come upon people like that who you don't understand what they're saying it almost seems like . . . you do feel bad because it almost seems like they humiliate you.

Another woman talked about the somatic symptoms she developed because she could not understand what people were saying to her, and she could not respond to them:

> The problem that I had was that when I would listen to people talk I would get a headache because I didn't understand, so my head would hurt a lot. When I would listen to people talk I would ask myself, what is this? What are they talking about?

The language barrier was not only a problem for these women when they initially immigrated, but continued to impact their lives at the time of the interview. Communication difficulties were especially problematic when they needed to access healthcare. Each of the women talked about how the CHA had helped them access the healthcare system whether by making appointments for them, accompanying them to appointments, or by helping them apply for services such as WIC (Women's Infant and Children's assistance) or public aid. "The health promoter helped me fill out the paperwork to apply for the medical card, also [she] helped me make the appointments," said a participant. One woman recalled, "The health promoter helped me to do such things as appointments because you [the health promoter] used to take me to those appointments where I didn't understand English, so you would help me with that."

Unfamiliarity with their neighborhood, the city, and the transportation system kept some of the women from getting the help they needed. One stated, "It's very hard for me to go to places by myself 'cause I feel like I'm going to get lost or something." Three of the women mentioned instances when the CHA had taken them to medical appointments. "She also helped me because she took me herself to the clinic."

> When I first met you [the health promoter], remember, I had a problem with my foot so you took me to get it treated at Cook County, but then I stopped going for the treatment because I got pregnant and so that's when you used to take me back and forth for whatever I needed for the pregnancy.

In one case it was spontaneously stated:

> Yes, she helped me, she showed me how to go to the places that I
> needed to go. She taught me how to get to these places so that by the
> next time I could go and do it by myself.

Even while transporting clients, the CHA did not simply serve as a chauffeur
for these women. She used the experience to teach them a new skill.

Three of the women identified specific instances when the CHA had
referred them to an agency or program that could further help them. Two were
referred to a food pantry at the health center where the CHA's office is located.
One spoke of the referral that the CHA made to a healthcare provider:

> The first thing that worried me the most was learning how to take care
> of my daughter and so that is when you helped me, you explained to
> me how to take care of a baby, how to help her get ahead, what kind of
> foods to give her. You took me to where they would explain to me
> how to take care of her.

Besides the referral, the CHA had provided a client with information about
available health resources so that the client could go to these resources when
she encountered problems herself or with members of her family.

All of the women stated that they had received some type of educational
information from the CHA. She helped one woman with beginning literacy
skills: "I learned a lot from you because you have taught me a lot of things like
how to write my name, because I didn't know how to do that."

As mentioned above, the CHA had taught some of the women how to use
public transportation so they could get to appointments or simply move about
in their community. One women remarked, "I've also learned how to get
around by myself. I learned also how to get around in the streets here, something that I didn't know before."

In terms of health education, the women stated that they had received a lot
of information from the CHA. Primarily she provided information about
public health concerns such as lead poisoning, nutrition, exercise, and immunizations. The health education that she gave was reflected in the following:

> I've also learned how to use a phone, how to express my needs or
> whatever I needed. I've even learned how to take better care of myself,
> what's good and bad. It's a different type of life in Mexico than the
> one we live here. Over here, we have learned more about my health,
> even how to take care of things in my house. Most of all I've also
> learned about cleanliness, how to keep the house clean; such things to
> be aware of, like lead, and to keep it free from insects. I feel that I've
> gotten a lot of very important information such as vaccinations; that
> it's very important for [kids] to get vaccinated in order for them to

grow up healthy. I also learned about lead, how to keep the kids free from getting lead. I didn't know anything about this before. Also I am better aware of health foods that we can eat, what kind of health foods for kids to eat, since they are little, to make a good start of healthy eating and to continue until they get big.

Another woman said that the CHA taught her how to breastfeed and how to take care of a sick baby. Still another related how the CHA had given her education about health promotion activities such as self-breast examination and exercise.

Characteristics of the CHA

The personal characteristics of the CHA as described by the women are summarized below. Apart from being knowledgeable, she was perceived by the women to be approachable and available.

All of the women stated that they appreciated the knowledge of the CHA. She was able to direct them to resources and teach them how to improve their health. Her knowledge of the healthcare system and how to access it was invaluable to these women because she provided a link between them and the larger system. One woman who had received help from the CHA in obtaining a Medicaid card said that, "The program is very good because the people that don't know how to get help from different places find out where they can get help and how to go about getting the help, such as obtaining a medical card." From their comments, it was evident that the participants depended on her to provide them with the help and answers they needed. According to one woman:

If I had the same problem again I would approach you to see what kind of advice you could give us about whatever problem we have. . . . Whenever we have any kind of health question we know that we can always ask her [the health promoter] because she can give us the answer.

Three of the women had been referred to the CHA by other family members or friends. One was referred by a clinic in the community, and another was referred through a health promoter in another community area. The referring parties viewed the CHA as someone who was available to help others. One woman's brother-in-law was working with the CHA and told her that the health promoter was "a very nice person" and would probably be able to help her with her financial and health problems.

One of the women related that she found the health promoter to be "very helpful and she's very nice. Also, because [she is] so patient, she doesn't lose her patience with us when we don't understand or we don't know things." The client was comfortable asking questions of the CHA, and the CHA made the client feel comfortable in approaching her with questions and concerns.

Since they find the CHA so approachable and knowledgeable, three of the women said that they had referred other friends and family members to her. They view her as a person who is able to help others. One woman stated:

> Well, you have helped everyone that's involved in my family and I've also seen that you have helped people that go there to approach you. I've seen you've helped people to get such things like food. I don't know their names [of the people that you've helped], but I know that I've seen them at the center where you've gotten a card to purchase things that they need.

All of the women indicated that they would contact the health promoter if they had problems in the future. This not only demonstrated their reliance on her, but also their belief that she would be available to them if they should need her. One woman said, "I feel better knowing she is here to help me when I need her; she's close by and I now know where the clinic is." Another commented, "Whenever I need help I go to the health promoter." One of the participants discussed how the health promoter's availability and dependability has made the health promoter their main resource for help: "We really don't know who to go to for any type of help except her [the health promoter] because she has always helped us . . . whenever [we] need something we know that we can count on someone here to help us."

Behavioral and Affective Responses of Client

The women cited examples of how they had been affected as a result of their interaction with the CHA. They reported that they had gained knowledge and were able to help others with what they had learned. In addition they came to rely on the CHA for assistance, and became more independent in some areas.

Each of the women stated that they learned many things from the CHA. Four of the five women directly linked their increased knowledge to their feelings of increased confidence and satisfaction. Some of their comments were:

> I now feel a little better because before, as you know, I didn't know much, I had a lot of questions for you and now I've learned more things.

And,

> I feel a lot more confident now. I feel like I am a different person even, because I know I have learned how to take care of a baby; I've also . . . learned how to take care of another person that's sick.

One of the women planned to build on her knowledge by attending a health promoter training session.

Another component of an increased sense of confidence among the women was that they told others about what they learned from the CHA. One women noted, "Yes, I have tried to [share] whatever I've learned, the little bit that I have learned. . . . I feel satisfied that whatever I have learned, I do share with others." Sharing information with family members and friends was a way the women could help others. "Although I don't know very many people here, we still, as far as [with] our family members, we talk to each other about what we've learned from [the health promoter]."

Each of the women said that one of the ways they helped others was by making referals to the health promoter. "I have tried also to help people by when they need something if I know where to tell them to get that help," said one of the participants. Another woman stated, "I help others through what I have learned. The way I help them is to recommend them to you [the health promoter] because you know more about these things."

As mentioned above, the women all came to value the CHA as a person who could help them and give them information to improve their health. Knowing they had a source of help gave these women a sense of confidence and security.

Four of the women said they thought it was important to be able to do things by themselves. However, they also discussed fear, shyness, and lack of knowledge as reasons why they were not able to be more independent. In spite of these barriers to independence, each woman mentioned examples of ways she had become more autonomous. The example cited by three women was their ability to navigate and to know how to get to their destinations.

DISCUSSION

When the data above are examined as aspects of empowerment as outlined by Walls (1996), the description of the women's growth can be assessed to see if it reflects actual empowerment.

It may not appear that the women in this study became empowered if empowerment is defined as independence and complete self-reliance. However, if empowerment is viewed as the benefits of an interdependent relationship, these women can be described as being empowered by their association with the CHA.

If the themes that emerged from these interviews are compared with the aspects of empowerment as outlined by Walls (Table 1), then these women became empowered. The primary means of empowerment for these women was their relationship with the CHA. Their participation and collaboration with their advocate resulted in a close and trusting relationship. In turn, they were able to mentor and form relationships with other people in their neighborhood. This is an outworking of the "train the trainee" concept.

Additional evidence of their empowerment was the experience and knowledge they gained. The new skills and information they learned was vital to the improvement of their sense of competency and well-being. Their ability to care for themselves and their families was enhanced. This may be especially significant for Hispanic women because they are the primary caregivers in their families and they are the principal link between their families and the larger healthcare system.

Furthermore, the women moved to a new level of self-knowledge. They became aware of their own capabilities; they found they were able to learn, grow, and adapt in a foreign, sometimes hostile, environment. They said they were able to overcome some of their fears.

Through their relationship with the CHA, they also attained a level of trust, both for themselves and for others. This trust was key in enabling them to be able to feel secure in their partnership with the CHA, and it made them feel comfortable in coming to the advocate with any concerns they had. The things they learned from the CHA made them feel more confident and capable as they interacted with people and institutions in their community.

The individual women were at different stages in terms of the amount of change they could tolerate, their motivation, and the realization of outcomes in their lives. For example, the woman who did not have literacy skills was more dependent on the CHA than the woman who was taking English classes. The CHA had developed a strong sense of the readiness and abilities of each woman. Although the advocate worked toward maximizing each woman's level of independence, the CHA viewed empowerment as a continuum. The advocate tailored her expectations and interventions to meet the needs of the individual woman. The CHA encouraged each one according to the level of empowerment each individual attained.

Further study using a quantitative methodology should be used to verify and generalize the findings of this project. A group receiving a healthcare intervention from a CHA could be compared with a group who did not participate in the program. A new or existing tool could be used to measure each participant's level of empowerment.

Another interesting area of inquiry would be a study of clients in the SLIAG program. Clients could be tracked throughout their time in the SLIAG program (or five to ten years) with periodic interviews and questionnaires to measure their level of empowerment. Data could be compared from the start to the end of the study to measure how the participants had become empowered and which interventions had been particularly beneficial.

According to the Hispanic immigrant women in this study, they became empowered through their relationships with the nurse/health advocate team. In light of this, community health nurses need to seek out, train, and collaborate with natural helpers within the community. These helpers can then become health advocates in the community, working along with community members to improve everyone's health. The health advocate takes on an especially important role in underserved communities, such as immigrant or low-income communities, because the people in these communities often are disconnected from each other and from the resources within their communities. The health advocate bridges this gap by placing herself in direct relationship with the individual needing care and then working with the individual toward improving his or her health. One of the women in the study stated:

Probably if you [the health promoter] hadn't taught me how to [go to the clinic], probably now I still wouldn't know how to do it or where to go. And so I've learned those type of things because of you. I feel more at ease now because, although I [still] don't know a lot, I have learned some things because of you, the things that you've taught me.

Through relationships of empowerment, individuals can move toward an increased sense of confidence and well-being. The empowering relationship between a CHA and individuals in the community can contribute to the improvement of the community's health as a whole.

REFERENCES

Barron, M. K. (1994). *Evaluation of a nurse/health advocate program for Hispanic immigrants: A primary healthcare intervention.* Unpublished master's thesis, University of Illinois at Chicago.

Bray, M. L., & Edwards, L. H. (1994). A primary health care approach using Hispanic outreach workers as nurse extenders. *Public Health Nursing, 11*(1), 7–11.

Caudle, P. (1991). Providing culturally-sensitive health care to Hispanic clients. *Nurse Practitioner, 18*(12), 40–51.

Chalmers, K., & Kristajanson, L. (1989). The theoretical basis for nursing at the community level: A comparison of three models. *Journal of Advanced Nursing, 14,* 569–574.

Clinton, B., & Lamer, M. (1988). Rural community women as leaders in health outreach. *Journal of Primary Prevention, 9*(1 and 2), 120–129.

Connelly, L. M., Keele, B. S., Kleinbeck, S. V. M., Schneider, J. K., & Cobb, A. K. (1993). A place to be yourself: Empowerment from the client's perspective. *IMAGE: Journal of Nursing Scholarship, 25*(4), 297–303.

Cottrell, L. S. (1976). The competent community. In B.H. Kaplan, R. N. Wilson, & A. H. Leighton (Eds.), *Further explorations in social psychiatry* (pp. 195–209). New York: Basic Books, Inc.

Eng, E., Salmon, M. E., & Mullen, F. (1992). Community empowerment: The critical base for primary health care. *Family and Community Health, 15*(1), 1–11.

Freire, P. (1993). *Pedagogy of the oppressed.* New York: Seabury.

Furino, A. & Mufioz, E. (1991). Health status among Hispanics: Major themes and new priorities. *JAMA, 265*(2), 255–257.

Gibson, C. H. (1991). A concept analysis of empowerment. *Journal of Advanced Nursing, 16,* 354–361.

Gonzales-Swafford, M. J., & Gutierrez, M. G. (1983). Ethno-medical beliefs and practices of Mexican Americans. *Nurse Practitioner, 6,* 29–34.

Israel, B. A. (1985). Social networks and social support: Implications for natural helper and community level interventions. *Health Education Quarterly, 12*(1), 65–80.

Juarbe, T. C. (1995). Access to health care for Hispanic women: A primary health care perspective. *Nursing Outlook, 43*(1), 23–28.

Keeney, G. B. (1993). *Access to health care; Barriers among an urban Hispanic immigrant community.* Unpublished master's thesis, University of Illinois at Chicago.

Knafl, K. A. & Webster, D. C. (1988). Managing and analyzing qualitative data. *Western Journal of Nursing Research, 10,* 195–218.

Leonard, V. (1989). A Heideggerian phenomenological perspective on the concept of the person. *Advances in Nursing Science, 11*(4), 40–55.

Lipson, J. G., McElmurry, B. J., & LaRosa, J. (1995). *Women across the lifespan: A working group on immigrant women and their health.* American Academy of Nursing, Washington, D. C.

Mahon, J., McFarlane, J., & Golden, K. (1991). De madres a madres: A community partnership for health. *Public Health Nursing, 8*(1), 15–19.

Maglacas, A. M. (1988). Health for all: Nursing's role. *Nursing Outlook, 36*(2), 66–71.

Mattson, M. T. (1990). *Atlas of the 1990 census.* New York: Macmillan Publishing Company.

May, K. M., Mendelson, C., & Ferketich, S. (1995). Community empowerment in rural health care. *Public Health Nursing, 12*(1), 25–30.

McElmurry, B. J., Swider, S. M., Bless, C., Murphy, D., Montgomery, A., Norr, K., Irvin, Y., Gantes, M., & Fisher, M. (1990). Community health advocacy: Primary health care nurse-advocate teams in urban communities. In *Perspectives in Nursing 1989–1991* (Publication Number 41-2281). New York, NY: National League for Nursing.

Meister, J. S., Warrick, L. H., de Zapien, J. G., & Wood, A. H. (1992). Using lay health workers: Case study of a community-based prenatal intervention. *Journal of Community Health, 17*(1), 37–51.

Minkler, M. (1992). Community organizing among the elderly poor in the United States: A case study. *International Journal of Health Services, 22*(2), 303–315.

Patton, S. (1995). Empowering women: Improving a community's health. *Nursing Management, 26*(8), 36–41.

Reinert, B. R. (1986). The healthcare beliefs and values of Mexican Americans. *Home Healthcare Nurse, 4*(5), 23–31.

Swider, S. M., & McElmurry, B. J. (1990). A woman's health perspective in primary health care: A nursing and community health worker demonstration project in urban America. *Family and Community Health, 13*(3), 1–17.

Walls, P. (1996). *Newman's theory and community participation in primary health care: The meaning of empowerment to persons.* Unpublished doctoral candidate's dissertation, Loyola University, Chicago.

Wilson, D. (1995). Women's roles and women's health: The effect of immigration on Latina women. *Women's Health Issues, 5*(1), 8–14.

Wilson, R. N. (1976). Editorial note to the competent community. In B. H. Kaplan, R. N. Wilson, & A. H. Leighton (Eds.), *Further explorations in social psychiatry* (pp. 193–194). New York: Basic Books, Inc.

Chapter 6

Issues in the Evaluation
of Primary Health Care Projects

KATHLEEN F. NORR
BEVERLY J. MCELMURRY

Dr. McElmurry was principal investigator and Dr. Norr was project evaluator on the Primary Health Care in Urban Communities project, funded by the Chicago Community Trust, the W. K. Kellogg Foundation, the Robert R. McCormick Charitable Trust, Illinois Department of Transportation, DHHS, Office of Minority Health, Blue Cross/Blue Shield, and the University of Illinois College of Nursing.

The tenets of Primary Health Care (PHC), first stated almost twenty years ago, have inspired numerous projects and healthcare system changes, and PHC has been credited with substantial improvements in health internationally. However, there are relatively few published evaluations of PHC projects and even fewer that are notable for their high quality. Factors contributing to this research gap include a paucity of funds for such evaluations and the relatively long time frame for results which make high-quality research difficult to conduct. In addition, we argue that the nature of the PHC model and the community context in which such projects occur present major conceptual, logistical, and ethical difficulties. None of these difficulties is unique to PHC research but their simultaneous presence makes evaluation of PHC projects especially challenging.

In this chapter, we describe our experience in evaluating a particular PHC demonstration project, the Primary Health Care in Urban Communities (PHCUC) project, implemented in Chicago from 1987 to 1993. We discuss the process of developing and implementing a PHC project in an inner-city environment. Building on these experiences, we identify key issues in the evaluation of PHC projects and possible strategies for addressing these issues as well as the lessons learned from our experience.

PLANNING THE PHCUC PROJECT EVALUATION

PHCUC Model

The definition of PHC provides a vision of what a healthcare system ought to be. However, there are no specific guidelines for moving from the existing system toward a PHC model. The major goal of the PHCUC project was to bring about collaboration between the healthcare system, the university, and the community around shared community health issues. We especially wanted to engage in a dialogue that would help community residents define and address their health concerns. We developed a conceptual model of how this process could be used through a new organizational structure: a team of nurses, trained community residents, and university-based support staff, who would work together to bridge the gap between the community, the healthcare system, and the university.[1]

PHC views health as an integral part of the overall social and economic development of a community. In inner-city, low-income communities many health problems are inseparable from economic and social issues such as poverty, poor housing, crime, and substance abuse, making a multi-sectoral approach to

---

[1]The conceptual basis and history of this model are described in greater detail in McElmurry et al. (1990); McElmurry, Swider, & Norr, (1991); and McElmurry & Newcomb (1995). Also, see Chapter 1 in this book.

health especially appropriate. However, the PHC model has rarely been used in industrialized countries or in urban areas. PHCUC was one of the first major demonstrations of the applicability of PHC to inner-city health problems in the United States. We planned to work in two communities, one predominantly African American and one predominantly Latino, where we had established a number of formal and informal ties. Both communities were plagued with all the problems of poverty, deteriorating neighborhoods, crime and violence, substance abuse, lack of education, and early childbearing common to inner-city and peri-urban communities worldwide.

The purpose of the PHCUC project was to demonstrate that a nurse-advocate-university support staff model could effectively address health issues collaboratively with the community. Although we knew what sort of community health promotion process we wanted to implement, we did not begin with a predetermined, specific set of health promotion activities. PHC as defined by the literature and by our model meant that specific health issues needed to be defined through genuine community collaboration. We did not intend to provide the type of primary care services found in clinics. Specific community health issues and activities were expected to emerge over time in collaboration with community residents, and these specific issues might be quite different in the two communities. Therefore, this demonstration project was evaluated primarily by the degree to which its process objectives were accomplished.

Developing a Framework for Evaluation

The conceptual model of the project dictated two defining characteristics for evaluation. First, the evaluation would focus primarily on documenting process and process-related outcomes, not on health outcomes specific to individuals or communities. Second, we saw the evaluation as an important component of the participatory and collaborative team we wanted to establish. While the university partners would contribute technical expertise in evaluation, the team as a whole would establish the objectives of the evaluation, participate in its implementation, and use results to reflect upon and improve the project. Additionally, we wanted the project evaluation to describe in detail the processes, procedures, and emerging roles of the public health nurse-advocate-university team to facilitate replication and document the effectiveness of this model for PHC in inner-city communities.

For our evaluation model, we adapted the framework of prospective analysis, a tool developed by the Pan-American Health Organization (PAHO) for participatory PHC initiatives. Prospective analysis is a strategy for helping groups envision what currently exists in healthcare and what they want to have in the future. The groups can then identify what needs to change to move toward their vision. This process was used by PAHO as a planning tool, not for evaluation. However, we felt that this approach provided a way to move from a general conceptual model to specific objectives which could then form a framework for planning evaluation.

Prospective analysis identifies four key areas to consider in projecting change: context, structure, function, and integrity. Once we collaboratively identified the major changes we wanted to see in each area, these became the component areas to be evaluated. **Context** refers to the initial environment, its challenges, resources, and major players. To address the context, our overall objective was to have project staff work collaboratively with community residents, agencies, and the university to identify health goals and resources in each community. **Structure** refers to the internal and external components that must emerge for success. Our primary objective was to establish an effective PHC team of nurses, health advocates, and university support staff. To do this required recruitment, training, and development of the roles of advocate, nurse-leader, and university-based support structures. **Function** refers to the efforts undertaken to achieve goals. The function objective of the PHCUC project was to work collaboratively with residents to address community health-related issues using nurse-advocate teams in two low-income communities. **Integrity** refers to the gradual development of linkages between the project and its environment to become part of the way things are done and to persist over time. Our objective was to establish linkages and cooperative activities among the health advocacy project, the community, health professionals, and the university that would promote community health and foster the continuation of a PHC model.

Implementing the Evaluation Plan

The evaluation used multiple data collection, analysis, and dissemination strategies to evaluate different aspects of the project and to meet different evaluation purposes. What was noteworthy about project implementation was not the techniques used but their participatory development and implementation. A primary focus of the project's participatory evaluation was to use the information about the project to generate insights about project challenges and accomplishments. This required the development of an ongoing analysis strategy with shared development of interpretations and meanings and feedback loops linking evaluation staff to project personnel.

One example of this collaborative evaluation process was the encounter form which the project used to document the advocate and nurse activities. Given the strong emphasis on quantitative outcome evaluation that dominates the public health field, we knew it was important to document numbers and types of nurse-advocate team activities. The evaluator and both teams had several meetings where we discussed the types of activities they did and the need to minimize record keeping in order to maximize team productivity. The evaluator used all this input to develop a one-page form for all types of activities that required minimal writing. After the advocates tried out the form, we met and revised it based on their experiences. The nurses and advocates recorded all the information about their activities, at first on paper and later on a computerized form.

Regular collective discussion and interpretation of the encounter forms provided a way for the team as a whole to reflect upon and improve the project and also promoted projectwide commitment to evaluation. Simple summaries were produced quarterly and discussed in staff meetings. We first became sensitized to the unique character of community mobilization activities when we realized that these activities were difficult to summarize adequately on the existing form. Subsequent discussion led to a revision of the form and helped deepen our understanding of community mobilization activities and their critical contribution to PHCUC goals. As advocates saw the documentation of their daily work, their perspective on record keeping began to change. Historically the advocates had few positive experiences with paperwork; they associated paperwork with negative feedback, bureaucratic encounters, and other obstacles they had experienced in the schools, public aid offices, or other healthcare facilities. Gradually they came to view record-keeping as a self-monitoring process that could contribute to project and personal growth.

DOCUMENTING PROJECT ACCOMPLISHMENTS

Context Outcomes

During the first year, the nurse-advocate teams interviewed residents, local leaders, and organizations and conducted a geographic survey of community resources (McElmurry et al., 1990). This process helped us understand the community context, established links between the nurse-advocate team, and community organizations and individuals, and began the process of collaboration to define and address health issues. Community information was then integrated with epidemiologic and census data compiled by university staff to develop a health issues assessment and a health resources directory for each community. A computerized database for all Chicago communities as well as the two assessments and resource directories were made available at the university and they were widely used by community leaders, health professionals, faculty, and students. Our collaboration with the communities around health issues continued to grow over time. Periodically we formally collaborated with residents to update community health priorities.

Structure Outcomes

The establishment of nurse-advocate teams supported by university staff, who worked collaboratively with the community to identify and address health issues, was the most important and most novel aspect of the project. Therefore, documenting how this organization was structured and operated was a critical part of the evaluation. After briefly describing the methods used to evaluate the structure, we will describe the nature of the organizational structure, roles, and relationships that emerged and the lessons learned about how to sustain such structures.

The evaluation strategies used to document and interpret the structure that emerged over time included: regular observation and participant observation of meetings and project activities, project records, in-depth interviews, focus groups with the advocates, and self-reflection and writing by the nurses and advocates. The evaluation of the training of health advocates used similar strategies and is described in Chapter 3 as well as in Swider & McElmurry (1990). Each of these strategies contributed a different perspective on the overall structure of the project. Observations focused on the way in which team members performed activities and related to other team members and to community residents and leaders. Individual and focus group interviews provided a time for nurses and advocates to explore their changing roles, relationships, and perceptions. In retrospect we realized we should have devoted more time to observation and interviews with the university staff.

The nurse-health advocate team was developed as the core organizational structure for delivering urban primary health care. In each of the two communities there was a team of one nurse and four to six health advocates established in their own office. At the university, the PHCUC project had offices and a large conference room with a support staff that included the part-time personnel of principal investigator, evaluator, community database manager, and one or more graduate research assistant(s), and the full-time support staff of project manager, secretary, and policy analyst (last two years only). Both nurse-advocate teams developed a regular weekly meeting for reaching consensus on activities and processing interpersonal and job performance issues. One nurse-advocate team devoted additional time to "gripe sessions" where personal conflicts were aired and resolved separately from work-related issues. The entire team met at the university site every other week.

When the program started, the advocate role was defined only in very general terms. The personal growth of the advocates over the course of the project was extraordinary. Most of them had never worked and had little hope of ever leaving public aid and public housing. Many went from being intimidated by presenting health education information in a small group to confidently going to the mayor's office or state legislature to offer testimony on a policy issue.

The nurses came to our project with extensive experience in community work and public health nursing. Thus, they had a role-model for how to be a nurse. However, they quickly discovered that being the nurse-leader of the PHC team was not like their previous roles. They eventually established a nurses support group to help them understand and process their experiences. Eventually, the nurses collaborated in publishing an article describing the multiple challenges of their roles as nurse-leaders and the different strategies they developed to deal with these challenges (Bless, Murphy, & Vinson, 1995).

The university support staff had a role model for what they would contribute based on extensive experience directing community health research and demonstration projects and had a role model for what they should contribute. They too discovered that this participatory project was not like their previous experience. The support staff provided a broader perspective on PHC, experience in establishing model programs, and overall leadership; technical expertise in health-related topics, evaluation, and dissemination; and resources and specific services, including connections to other institutions and organizations, fiscal management, and access to university services and facilities.

The PHCUC project operated in a participatory and consensual style. This was both a major accomplishment of the project and a continuing challenge to implement and maintain. Throughout the project, we tried to foster working relationships that were collaborative and empowering and thus congruent with the way the teams were expected to work with the community and the university. Over time, these working relationships strengthened the advocates' effectiveness through personal growth and gradually increasing autonomy. Decision making sought to integrate the perspectives of all team participants while simultaneously taking advantage of the special technical and policy experiences of university staff. For example, the team as a whole would come to consensus about major evaluation topics and the implications for the project of specific evaluation findings, but the evaluator would assume responsibility for technically correct data management, analysis, and presentation.

There were three somewhat interrelated barriers to a consensual style that had to be overcome. The first barrier, inherent in the participatory-consensual style, is that full participation and reaching consensus on important issues requires considerably more time in discussion and decision making than either a bureaucratic or majority rule management style. The large size of the total group was a factor that made reaching consensus slow and difficult.

A second challenge was the diversity of the PHCUC team, a characteristic that both strengthened the quality of consensual decisions and made reaching consensus a more complex and time-consuming process. The considerable gulf between the university staff, nurses, and advocates in life experiences, education, values, and work habits made team-building especially challenging. The advocates had a more holistic approach to relationships. For them, work relationships were subordinate to a judgment of the person, especially regarding respect for others, loyalty, and trustworthiness. However, once they did accept a new team member they were quite tolerant of personal differences and they extended trust across the board. The professionals, both nurses and university support staff, did much more compartmentalization in their relationships (e.g., work versus social, good at telephone contacts but not good at group classes). The nurses had a practice orientation that was less concerned with theory and more concerned with concrete accomplishments. The university staff had a tendency to dominate the agenda and discussion during staff meetings. The traditional educational background and inclinations of the academically based staff valued abstract thought, generalization, and compartmentalization of feelings and relationships. This style was in direct opposition to the more concrete and holistic thinking and relationship styles of the advocates. The nurses often found themselves quite literally in the middle, trying to act as interpreters and brokers between these two worlds. Given the participatory approach embedded in a PHC philosophy, this challenge of bridging diverse cultures is an ongoing challenge but one well worth the investment in time, energy, and critical reflection.

Developing a cohesive and effective team that integrated all these diverse life experiences and relational styles required a great deal of effort and a common commitment to the project's model. One of the critical strategies for consensus building was making sure that university-based staff got out into the communities and met frequently with the nurse-advocate teams in their setting. Although such visits were short, they had a profound educative impact in helping staff understand the advocate perspective and experience of the community.

A third barrier was the bureaucratic structures within which the PHCUC project was embedded currently, as well as the prior experiences of all the participants. The bureaucratic environment of the university set limits on the sharing of responsibility and required conformity to some bureaucratic standards such as the fiscal reporting and inflexible work rules for nonfaculty employees. This made the principal investigator the head of the project and the nurse the "boss" of the nurse-advocate team, which partially conflicted with their participatory leadership roles. The nurses especially felt a great deal of pressure to ensure that the team conformed to regulations and was productive.

A more general problem was the pervasiveness of noncollegial models of decision making. The nurses and the advocates had very little familiarity with a collaborative or collegial work structure and a great deal of familiarity with bureaucratic, top-down structures and leadership styles. The academic staff in the university setting had somewhat more familiarity with collegial consensus-based decision making, but they were not accustomed to an environment where their scholarly insights and technical skills had to be expressed effectively to nonexperts and were just one component to be considered in decision making.

On the whole, the project was remarkably successful in achieving consensual decision making on major project issues and on gradually establishing a balance of power between the nurse-advocate teams and university staff. There were times of heated debate about policy and project alternatives that took a toll on interpersonal relationships. While we almost always succeeded in finding a course that was at least acceptable to all, we sometimes resented the time that it took to do so, especially the more time-sensitive university staff. Reaching consensus for decisions seemed to work better within the nurse-advocate teams. They were smaller, had a more equitable balance of power, and spent more time together. Although the nurse had higher status and more formal power, there were four to five advocates at the same level so that they found the nurse less intimidating. By the end of the project the nurse-advocate teams were actively setting their own future directions for development and sharing efforts to obtain funding.

For the PHCUC team, acquiring firsthand knowledge of the community and individual struggles and challenges created stress and sorrow. These feelings were especially challenging for the advocates. As they gained greater understanding and new perspectives, they had to develop new ways of viewing their community, their neighbors, and their own lives. The university staff also experienced a great deal of stress in trying to interpret the project to their colleagues in the privileged world of the university. The nurse-advocate teams

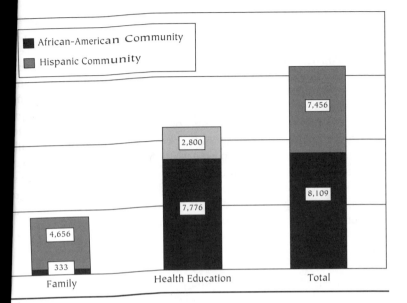

1.
f persons directly served by the PHCUC project health workers

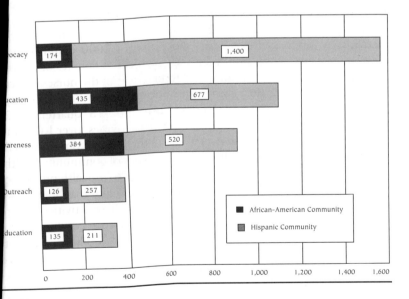

RE 2.
er and type of PHCUC activities

worked in close proximity and many interpe
be resolved. It took a long time for relatic
develop, and it was only after trust was estab
be truly collaborative. Addressing these em
focus of team building, and required far more
inally anticipated. We eventually developed re
the advocates with a community psycholog
nurses. We also provided ongoing continuii
advocates, together and separately, that both e
team members broaden their perspectives and
supported advocates who wanted to go back to
cates completed junior college or college while
ever, no supports were in place for the university
be given more attention in future projects.

20,000

15,000

10,000

5,000

0

Function Outcomes

The **function** objective of engaging in activities
issues was the easiest aspect of the PHCUC proj
to use the data the nurse-advocate teams genera
and types of nurses-advocate team activities. This
quarters (3.25 years). The form was not used du
six months devoted mainly to dissemination. Qua
advocate activities provided insights into how the
how they interacted with community members ar
strengths and limitations of their efforts.

The nurse-advocate teams' records of their wor
ductivity. In just over three years, more than 15,
received direct services from the PHCUC project as
health promotion groups (Figure 1). Observation of
ties identified some of the special contributions of t
pared to existing services. Encounter forms for
documented over 2,800 specific health-related activiti
can-American community and over 1,700 in the Latir
These activities encompassed three different types of c
tion: advocacy for 1,400 individual families, over 675
ties for groups, and over 750 community-wide activitie
mobilized residents around health issues. Most of these
than one contact: an average of 1.7 contacts per group
per family, and over 3 contacts per networking and mol

Advocacy for families meant helping them with a w
Many families had more than one concern, with an averag
per family. We classified the major issues of families accordi
Organization (WHO) eight essential elements of primar
slightly to fit the context of an urban industrialized coun

FIGURE
Number o

Family Ad

Health Ed

Raising Aw

Continuing

FIGU
Numb

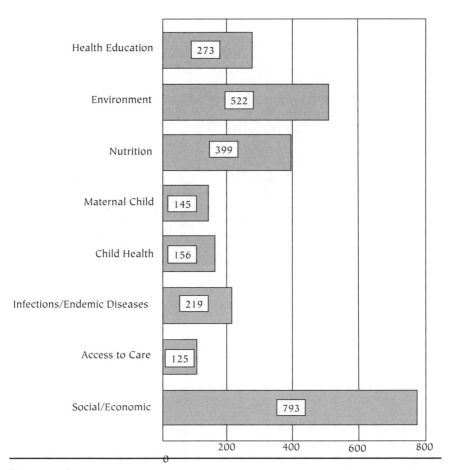

FIGURE 3.
Problems addressed in family advocacy
(November 1988 to January 1992)

WHO essential elements, environmental needs such as unsafe housing, nutrition, and lack of food were the most common problems. We had to add a category for other social and economic problems such as need for job skills, isolation, familial conflict, and anxiety. Almost a third of the families' concerns fell into this category.

The nurse-advocate teams offered a wide variety of health education sessions, support groups, and health screening related to health issues identified by people in the community (Figure 4). About a quarter of these activities focused on specific health skills including first aid for children and cardiopulmonary resuscitation (CPR), requested especially by residents of high-rise public housing units where paramedics would not enter until police arrived. Another quarter of the activities focused on parenting, including parenting support groups. The advocates' parenting support groups were so highly

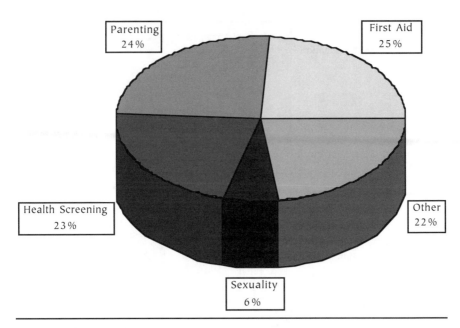

FIGURE 4.
Types of health education and screening groups
(November 1988 to January 1992)

regarded that the city's child protective services agency referred some parents and even made the class attendance a condition for regaining custody of their children for parents involved in neglect or abuse.

Observation showed that the nurse-advocate team provided family advocacy and group education in a style that was consistent with PHC emphasis on accessibility, acceptability, and participation. They increased accessibility by serving residents in naturally occurring community gathering places such as schools and churches or their homes rather than making the community come to them. The nurse-advocate team enhanced acceptability by adapting their message to the learning style, culture, and situations of people in the community. They emphasized participation, active learning, and effective use of community examples that were close to home. For families struggling to meet their needs in a fragmented health and welfare system, the advocate acted as a bridge between the client and services: explaining the healthcare and social welfare agency "culture" to the clients and explaining client needs and perspectives to the agencies.

The advocates' ability to rethink standard health education materials to make them more culturally sensitive and relevant was especially strong. For example, when the advocates decided to develop community programs on domestic violence they recognized from personal experience that many women went through a relatively lengthy process in getting ready to leave a violent situation. Current programs had nothing to offer these women about how to make their current situation safer or how to plan for leaving. This issue generated a great deal of debate within the project, with all the professional staff extremely reluctant to put anything in the program that might seem to support staying in a violent situation and the advocates vehemently insisting that these women needed concrete help with the realities they faced. Together, the staff developed a program that integrated strong support for leaving a violent situation with concrete advice about what to do while getting ready to leave.

Evidence of the participatory nature of both family and group advocacy activities comes from the way in which the two teams adapted their activities to the two different communities. Although the two nurse-advocate teams both reached approximately the same number of residents in direct services, the African-American community team focused mainly on health education and screening while the team in the Latino community provided much more advocacy to individual families. These differences reflected the different needs of the communities. In the African-American community, residents and outsiders were more fearful of entering unfamiliar areas or crossing gang boundaries and more wary of outsiders and new programs. The nurse-advocate team site was not accessible to the majority of residents because of gang boundaries or other barriers. This kept the residents from seeking out individualized services, but they were eager for health promotion in groups in safe areas of the community. In the Latino community, residents and outsiders felt safer moving about in the community, but there were many recent non-English-speaking immigrants who especially needed help in negotiating unfamiliar healthcare and social welfare systems. The nurse-advocate team was located in a primary care clinic where families coming for healthcare, and health professionals, often turned to the advocates to help address family health-related problems. Thus, family advocacy became a more important part of the work of the nurse-advocate team in the Latino community.

Over time, the nurse-advocate teams fostered team members' special skills and activities. One concern for the PHCUC project was having the capacities to address all the health issues the community identified. A small team of advocates and a nurse cannot be "experts" in everything, and probably should not try to be. Without developing a formal policy, informal ways of addressing this issue emerged. Advocates developed specialties that matched their particular interests and skills. Programs or activities that were widely accepted in the community were expanded while less popular activities ceased. This was not always efficient; the advocates often trained and invested energy in a particular activity and then abandoned it.

Later, the project agreed upon an overall focus on violence. Initially, both communities identified violence as the number one health issue, but in the beginning the nurse-advocate teams did not see any ways they could address this problem. Two years later, both teams began to identify violence reduction strategies. In the Latino community, they focused on domestic violence. In the

African-American community they provided a safe place for youths to meet as an alternative to being on the streets. Thus, a natural focus gradually emerged that united the communities' primary health concern and the advocates unique capacities.

Integrity Outcomes

The PHCUC project achieved substantial integration into the university, healthcare system, and communities. Activities that promoted integrity of the project and the environment were on three different levels: mobilization around health issues within the community, representation of community health issues to agencies and policy makers outside the community, and linking the project to others within the university. These activities were documented by quantitative data from the encounter forms, project records, news media coverage, observations of project activities, and interviews with university faculty involved in the training program.

The nurse-advocate teams worked with community organizations, public agencies and other groups to promote the PHCUC model and facilitate the process of identification of community health needs and the mobilization of resources to address those needs. The nurse-advocate teams participated in over 500 activities that increased public awareness of community health needs. They established collaborative working relationships with over 200 organizations, including other community organizations, local schools and churches, local and national healthcare-related organizations, government agencies, and the university.

Within the communities, the nurse-advocate teams participated in numerous collaborative activities and established ties with many community-based organizations. This integration into the structure of the community facilitated the nurse-advocate team efforts and made them better able to mobilize the community around health issues. For example, the Chicago Department of Health was using mobile vans to go into the community and immunize children, but these efforts did not bring out a large number of residents. When the advocates began going with the vans and knocking on doors to bring out residents, the number served increased dramatically. (See Figure 5.)

The advocate teams represented the health needs of inner-city communities in a wide variety of forums, including the City of Chicago's Health Summit, testimony before the state legislature, and workshops on PHC for health professionals. The PHCUC project developed and conducted two important local conferences, one on PHC and one on violence reduction for minority male adolescents. Both conferences were notable for their inclusion of local groups, health providers, agencies, and university members. The domestic violence brochures prepared by the advocates were adopted by the city department of health in 1996 and translated into many languages for use throughout the city.

The PHCUC project also developed many ties within the university. Over 30 faculty participated in the advocate training sessions and/or visited the

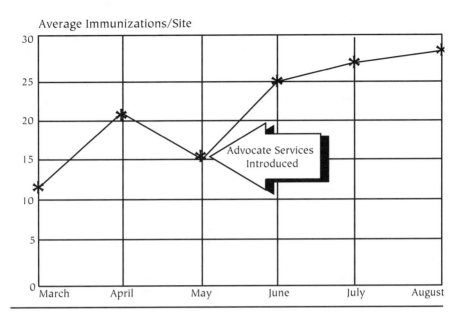

FIGURE 5.
Carevan immunizations in public housing sites
(1992 Carevan service)

project sites. In a survey conducted by a nonproject member, many of these faculty reported that participation in the project had stimulated them to integrate the concepts of PHC into their teaching and research. Undergraduate and graduate students in nursing, public health, medicine, dentistry, and the social sciences participated in internships with the PHCUC project. Also, the advocates were invited to speak about their work to several undergraduate and graduate level courses in nursing, their presentations were well received by both faculty and students.

As we gained experience in the PHCUC project, we gradually realized the importance and difficulty of community mobilization. The nurse-advocate teams started out most interested in providing direct health promotion and education services to families and community groups. As their community linkages and understanding of local health issues grew, they gained a greater appreciation of the importance of community mobilization and their capacity to provide leadership in mobilization and policy change.

Community mobilization activities require a huge and unpredictable time commitment, extensive networking and attendance at numerous meetings. The outcomes of these activities are much less predictable, less under the control of the project, and more likely to fail. Despite these obstacles, community mobilization remains a core concern for PHC, and it is essential to encourage and support these efforts. It is critical to help the community identify factors that relate to community health issues and then mobilize to improve their situation. Many community health problems require action on multiple levels to achieve a higher level of community wellness. Violence in the home is a typical example, requiring job training for women and legal changes as well as individual health education and support. A major strength of the PHC model is the capacity to link health with development and to focus on root causes of health issues.

DISCUSSION OF EVALUATION ISSUES

Collaborative Process

Developing and implementing an evaluation plan for this demonstration project presented several serious challenges to conventional evaluation strategies. Because the main objective of the PHCUC project was to initiate a collaborative process, we decided that the primary evaluation of project success should focus on the degree to which specific collaborative process objectives were achieved. Those who do not accept this will not accept our evaluation strategy. There remains a pervasive bias, especially in the healthcare field, in favor of outcome measures, preferably quantifiable and easily measured. Process evaluation has been used primarily for program development and description, not as an outcome measure. Rifkin, Muller, and Bichmann (1988) developed process outcomes to assess the degree of participation in PHC projects, but this approach has not been widely replicated. Likewise, research models that focus more on the collaborative process, such as action research and participatory research, have generally not been widely accepted into the mainstream of either evaluation or behavioral science methodology.

We would have liked to also evaluate community health outcomes, because the long-term desired outcome from this project was improved community health. A longitudinal study that examines changes in intervention and control communities' health status is one strategy for doing so. However, as Feinleib (1996) has recently pointed out, this approach is expensive, lengthy, and technically difficult. Several recent large community-based health promotion studies have failed to provide clear-cut results. The other commonly used strategy is to examine intermediate outcome objectives, such as "infant immunization rates will be increased by 50 percent," compared to baseline data or a matched comparison community. However, this approach requires prior collaboration with the community in defining health issues or, as is more often the case, eliminates the possibility of community participation at this important first stage. When specific health outcome objectives are defined through a collaborative process and are expected to be different for different communities, this approach becomes difficult and costly to implement. This would have required collection of a wide variety of health information when only a few would have been relevant. We decided that neither of these two ways to examine health outcomes for a demonstration project was feasible.

Evaluation Challenges of Community Collaboration

Community collaboration requires reconceptualizing the impact or effectiveness outcomes of a demonstration program is. Evaluation designs are usually built around an attempt to document as clearly as possible the unique impact of the project. However, a major goal of the PHCUC team was to work on health issues through collaboration with community organizations and residents. Collaborative activities cannot be attributed solely to project staff, yet most of them would not have occurred without the PHCUC project's efforts. Collaboration may also increase the collaborating organization's involvement in community health issues. This synergistic increase in community mobilization toward improving health is exactly the process the PHCUC project sought to initiate. In our opinion, the conventional approach to evaluation emphasizes identifying direct project impacts independent of other changes. This is not only technically difficult, but conceptually inappropriate for collaborative projects.

In community-based projects the evaluator needs to conduct the evaluation in a way that sustains collaboration. People and organizations in the community are often justifiably resentful of past research projects that have not incorporated the community perspective or helped to work toward solutions. In the PHCUC project these attitudes were also shared by the advocates, who came from the community. Thus, part of the role of the project evaluator is to show to community residents and organizations that evaluation can contribute to the project and the community.

Equally important is a sensitivity to the effects on the community of evaluation. While the evaluation must present a truthful picture of what has happened, analysis must be presented in a productive, consensus-building manner rather than an antagonistic or win/lose approach. Conventional mechanisms to safeguard confidentiality may be inadequate in a local community, and this will magnify the harmful effect of any negative evaluation.

Participatory Evaluation

At the onset of this project, none of the university-based staff had significant firsthand experience with collaborative evaluation. We had all been trained in traditional qualitative and quantitative research methodologies. Although action research and participatory research methodology provide a guiding framework for what a collaborative evaluation should be and how to organize such an endeavor (e.g., Brown & Tandon, 1983; Cousins & Earl, 1992), we only became aware of these models after the evaluation plan was developed (Feuerstein, 1986).

There are many costs to participatory evaluation. Different contributors have different perspectives, values, and interests that may lead them to perceive and evaluate the same situation differently. The process of trying to achieve consensus can disrupt working relationships and absorb time and energy. With more persons involved, the cost of coordination and training and the potential for errors increase. Moving toward a participatory model of evaluation has been a real challenge both for the more academic members of the team, who had to give up accustomed control over evaluation activities, and for the community-based advocate teams, who initially distrusted evaluation as threatening and/or a waste of time and money.

Many of the same factors that make participatory evaluation difficult to implement also increase the evaluation's validity and empower program participants (Hill, Bone, & Butz, 1996). Evaluation requires different perspectives and multiple talents difficult to find in one person but more likely to be present in a team. Incorporating evaluation into regular project activities means that broad coverage can be achieved within the project's time and money limitations. Participation in evaluation empowers project staff by giving them new perspectives and skills. Specifically, using evaluation to assess whether the project's activities are meeting goals mirrors the reflective problem-solving process that is central to PHCUC-community collaboration. As Weiss (1983) observes, participation in evaluation does not guarantee that evaluation results will be used. However, involving the entire team in evaluation remains one of the best ways to ensure that the project makes use of evaluation outcomes.

The scientifically most compelling advantage of participatory evaluation is its enhancement of validity. The involvement of community residents, and especially the health advocates, enhances both the quality of the information collected and interpretation of its meaning. Because the advocates were familiar with the community, they helped us gain safe access to areas, groups, and discussion topics that would normally be closed to us. They also helped us to bridge the wide gulf between the academic professional and the low-income resident. Valid interpretation is hampered by cultural differences, language barriers, and occasional deception. The advocates helped us arrive at a deeper understanding of what residents were really telling us and what project activities and accomplishments meant in the context of the community. Thus, collaboration fosters an interpretation that is grounded in both the philosophy of science and the lived experiences of community residents.

How much funding should be appropriated for evaluation of demonstration projects? Many funding agencies want to fund quality management activities appropriate for routine service delivery. Often, tension exists within project staff between the desire for a full and convincing evaluation and the desire to commit more resources to direct services. However, if a demonstration project seems successful, there is an urgent need for evidence of effective outcomes. Early in the project the evaluator must help the project team and funders to appreciate the benefits of systematic evaluation.

Evaluator's Role

Our experience in the PHCUC project was that directing a truly collaborative evaluation would be nearly impossible for an evaluator external to the project. Understanding the philosophy of the project was critical to the development of an evaluation plan for it. Establishing a trusting relationship was an essential first step in overcoming fear and resistance to evaluation among project staff. The evaluator also had to learn to trust the other project participants as evaluation partners. The degree of collaboration in evaluation gradually increased along with the growth of the project, as the academic support staff grew in their understanding of the capacities of the nurse-advocate teams and how to work effectively in partnership with them. We believe that it is very difficult to achieve this level of collaboration with an external evaluator.

In making decisions about the evaluation and its interpretation, the evaluator has unique technical knowledge and an understanding of the kind of evaluation data that can be persuasive to relevant audiences of health professionals, academics, politicians, and funders. The evaluator's job is to translate this knowledge into a form that can be understood by the team members and the community without taking over the decision-making process. We have come to realize that the evaluator's role in collaborative evaluation parallels the role of the advocate in the PHC team. Just as the advocate acts as a bridge between the health professional and the community, the evaluator must be a bridge between the PHC team and the community of evaluators.

L E S S O N S   L E A R N E D

The nurse-advocate team is a powerful model to achieve participatory PHC in inner-city American communities. Over a five-year period the PHCUC project succeeded in establishing two nurse-advocate teams in two very different inner-city communities. Both teams worked with community residents to define health issues and provide services that addressed the health concerns of the community. The model became popular with services providers and local organizations, many of whom incorporated aspects of the model into their programs. The model was very influential at the university, leading both the PHCUC university staff and others to develop new programs using the nurse-advocate team approach, as well as placing more emphasis on PHC concepts in course work.

The university is an important partner in PHC. In 1984, the WHO stated that universities had an important role to play in PHC by providing a repository of technical expertise, training opportunities, and as a "community of solutions;" however, few universities in industrialized countries have responded to this call for leadership. The PHCUC project has demonstrated that a team of university-based health professionals, educators, and researchers can provide leadership to sustain a nurse-advocate team working collaboratively in the community. The university staff played a critical role in all of the areas identified by WHO, including sharing of technical expertise in team organization, and health promotion content, evaluation, presentation, and publication. The university staff provided a role-model for collaborative team relationships with shared decision making, mutual respect, effective conflict resolution, and problem solving to generate creative solutions.

Equally important, providing leadership in a PHC demonstration project made major contributions to both participating faculty and the university. The participating faculty gained understanding of the applicability of PHC to urban health issues and enhanced their capacities to work collaboratively with community residents. For the university, PHC projects added to the collective intellectual capacities and resources and strengthened the education of health professionals for the changing context of healthcare today. Connections to the community also enhanced the relevance and contributions of the university, which in turn helped to justify continued public investment in universities. The PHCUC project and other PHC projects promote the university's transmission of civic values, especially the values of respect for cultural diversity and the valuing of an ethic of public service.

New activities in PHC programs should build upon team skills. Ideally, a PHC project responds to health issues that are defined by the community. However, a small team of advocates and a nurse cannot be experts in everything; nor should they have to be. Thus far we do not have sufficient experience with urban PHC programs to establish guidelines for how broad or narrow project activities should be.

As described earlier, the activities of the PHCUC project became more focused over time. The advocates developed areas of expertise that drew upon their interests and skills, so that not all members of the team performed the same activities. Eventually, a natural focus on violence reduction emerged that united the communities' health concerns and the nurse-advocates unique capabilities.

Community mobilization and policy initiatives are essential components of PHC programs. The PHC approach is more than providing services that meliorate health problems in the community through family advocacy or group health promotion and education. Although theses direct services are important because they help individuals and families and build credibility of the PHC team, it is essential that community residents identify health issues and interventions that they are willing to invest their time and energy in implementing. Most community health problems are multifaceted and require action on many levels to realize the goals of community wellness. For example, inner-city children are more likely to be incapacitated by asthma and to die from the disease. A multifaceted approach would provide not only services for asthmatic children, but would educate families, teachers, and health professionals about asthma management and implement strategies to reduce environmental factors, such as insect infestations, auto and industrial pollution, and irritants in homes.

At the onset of the PHCUC project, the nurse-advocate teams were more invested in providing direct health promotion and educational services to families. However, as their understanding of local health issues grew and community linkages expanded, the team gained an appreciation of the importance of community mobilization, took more leadership in mobilizing grassroots efforts, and strategized to effect broader changes in health policy. As the team's confidence and expertise grew they were no longer satisfied to only ameliorate health problems; instead they expanded their vision of community health to include approaches that impacted local and societal perceptions of health, as well as the social and political structures that directly affect community health.

Positive outcomes do not guarantee sustainable PHC programs. As Weiss (1986) observed more than a decade ago, whether a demonstration project is sustained depends upon many economic and political factors, so that a positive evaluation is usually necessary but never sufficient for sustainability. A major strength of the PHCUC model was its holistic approach to health issues which challenged the views of conventional healthcare systems, social agencies, and the university. However, a demonstration project by itself can have only a modest impact on the healthcare system as a whole. In the United States the healthcare system is still dominated by the medical model and primary care is often viewed as equivalent to PHC.

Long-run sustainability of a PHC program requires either that the healthcare system moves closer toward a PHC model or that the project is able to find some niche in the existing system where it can survive. The major social and economic issues that perpetuate inequality in access to healthcare and that block communities from achieving the level of health essential for development are also obstacles to PHC innovations. While the PHCUC project was able to attract sizeable levels of foundation funding for a demonstration project, foundations were unwilling to continue funding long enough to achieve long-term agendas.

CONCLUSION

Although the PHCUC project did not continue beyond the original funding period, this project stimulated many subsequent projects that all build on the PHCUC model of nurse-advocate teams to work on health issues in collaboration with the community (see Chapter 1). Nearly all of these subsequent projects have been more narrowly focused. Some have addressed a specific set of health issues, such as the REACH-Futures project on infant health promotion. Others have focused on the health issues of a more narrowly defined community, such as the PHC for Urban Children project which serves children and their families in a particular school. Still others have focused on education to increase the capacities for PHC collaboration of both health professionals and community residents, such as the Leadership Project and the Chicago Health Corps.

There is growing awareness in nursing and other health professions that the current healthcare delivery system has failed to provide adequate health promotion in the United States and has resulted in highly inequitable treatment of disease. New ways of delivering care must be developed, implemented, and evaluated. The PHC model provides one vision of how health professions, universities, and communities can collaborate around health issues, and the

PHCUC project demonstrated that this model can be implemented in our most impoverished communities. The evaluation of the PHCUC project was able to document these accomplishments, and confirms the importance of committing adequate resources for the evaluation of PHC projects.

REFERENCES

Bless, C., Murphy, D., & Vinson, N. (1995). Nurses' role in primary health care. *N&HC: Perspectives on Community, 16*(2), 70–76.

Brown, L. D., & Tandon, R. (1983). Ideology and political economy in inquiry: Action research and participatory research. *Journal of Applied Behavioral Science, 19*(3), 277–294.

Cousins, J. B., & Earl, L. M. (1992). The case for participatory evaluation. *Educational Evaluation and Policy Analysis, 14*(4), 397–418.

Feinleib, M. (1996). Editorial: New directions for community intervention studies. *American Journal of Public Health, 86*(12), 1696.

Feuerstein, M. T. (1986). *Partners in Evaluation*. London: Macmillan Education.

Hill, M. N., Bone, L. R., & Butz, A. M. (1996). Community-health workers in research. *Image: Journal of Nursing Scholarship, 28*(3), 221–226.

McElmurry, B. J., & Newcomb, B. J. (1995). Graduate nursing concentration in women's health at the University of Illinois at Chicago. *Health Care for Women International, 16*, 491–500.

McElmurry, B. J., Swider, S. M., Bless, C., Murphy, D., Montgomery, A., Norr, K., Irvin, Y., Gantes, M., & Fisher, M. (1990). Community health advocacy: Primary health care nurse-advocate teams in urban communities. In *Perspectives in nursing 1989–1991* (pp. 117–131). New York: National League for Nursing.

McElmurry, B. J., Swider, S. M., & Norr, K. (1991). A community-based primary health care program for integration of research, practice, and education. In *Curriculum revolution: Community building and activism* (pp. 77–90). New York: National League for Nursing Press.

Rifkin, S. B., Muller, F., & Bichmann, W. (1988). Primary health care: On measuring participation. *Sociology in Medicine, 26*(9), 931–940.

Swider, S. M., & McElmurry, B. J. (1990). A women's health perspective in primary health care: A nursing and community health worker demonstration project in urban America. *Family and Community Health, 13*(3), 1–17.

Weiss, C. H. (1983). Toward the future of stakeholder approaches in evaluation. In A. S. Bryk (Ed.), *Stakeholder-based evaluation* (pp.83–96). San Francisco: Jossey-Bass.

World Health Organization (1984). *The role of universities in the strategies for Health for All*. Geneva: WHO.

Chapter 7

Nurse/Health Advocate Team Model in Hispanic Immigrant Communities in Chicago

CHANG GI PARK
VIRGINIA WARREN
with the assistance of
RANDY SPREEN PARKER
BEVERLY J. MCELMURRY
CYNTHIA TYSKA

Project Design and Implementation:
Beverly J. McElmurry, principal investigator; Gwen Brumbaugh Keeny, research assistant; Aaron Busch, nursing supervision and case management; Ada Gonzalez, nursing supervision and case management; Martha Gonzalez, community health advocate; Celia Martinez, community health advocate.

Project Funding:
This project was partially funded by the Chicago Department of Public Health, the Coalition for Hispanic Health, and the State Legalized Immigration Assistance Grant (SLIAG). SLIAG was supported in part by the Chicago Health Coalition through a demonstration grant, D52-MP91161-01-1, from the Office of Minority Health and the University of Illinois at Chicago, College of Nursing.

HISTORY

In the summer of 1991, the Primary Health Care in Urban Communities (PHCUC) project of the University of Illinois at Chicago (UIC), College of Nursing, responded to a request from the Chicago Department of Public Health (CDPH) for proposals to address health issues of immigrants. Federal funding, the State Legalization Assistance Grant (SLIAG), became available to states and cities with significant immigrant populations to offset the cost of providing healthcare and social services to those newly legalized under the immigration Reform Act of 1986. A portion of Chicago's grant, administered by the CDPH and known simply by its acronym, SLIAG, was made available to community agencies, institutions, and organizations already providing health and social services to immigrant populations in Chicago. Federal funding for the program ended in 1996; however, recognizing its impact on Chicago's ethnic communities, CDPH has continued to sustain the program, now called "Door to Door," until 1998.

Since 1984, the PHCUC program has trained and deployed registered nurse/community health advocate (RN/CHA) teams as a key strategy for developing urban health education and promotion programs consistent with the primary health care (PHC) philosophy. For the SLIAG project, an RN and CHA work side-by-side to identify immigrant families and individuals needing health and social services, to evaluate and link them with local resources. The target population for this project is primarily Mexican, but also includes immigrants from Central and South America, and the Caribbean.

New immigrants to inner-city communities often live in isolation with few friends and little social support from the community. Accordingly, these families are hard to locate and connect with health and social services. Most have little or no understanding of the healthcare and social services system in the United States, and experience economic, linguistic, and cultural barriers to the access of needed services. Their health issues are, for the most part, those of a young population who have primarily preventable or curable health problems with early detection, health education, and access to primary care and social services. Nevertheless, access to health services is becoming increasingly difficult for immigrants due to the fragmented service delivery system. The special needs of immigrants combined with the structural limitations of the system create a situation that hinders the health and well-being of this target population.

PROGRAM CONCEPTS

The annual program objectives for each participating organization were: (1) Identify one hundred high-risk families, (2) assess the families and link them with health and social services in the community, (3) follow the families for one year to evaluate impact, and (4) increase the capacity of collaborating organizations to link and refer clients to community resources. Immigrants are likely to have difficulty in finding health and social services without the knowledge of local resources and the skills to gain access, and they are less likely to address their health needs in a timely and effective manner. Further, a community's capacity to provide health services for immigrants requires local health agencies to be responsive to their health needs. An effective program for meeting these objectives must view health, social, and economic problems as inseparable.

The PHCUC team complemented the goals of the CDPH with PHC strategies by expanding the program's scope. The roles of the nurse and CHA were implemented to increase the long-term effectiveness of the program. PHC strategies require that basic health needs are met with resources that are accessible, acceptable, and affordable to the community in a manner that ensures health maintenance activities are sustainable over time. Families and individuals know their health needs better than anyone else and are their own best resource. As active participants with local care and service providers, community residents are better equipped to address their health needs.

The project goal was to assist families to gain greater control over their health and well-being through a family-focused, community-based approach. The project objectives are as follows:

a. Identify families and individuals at risk through assertive outreach
b. Assess the individual and family's health needs whenever possible in the home
c. Promote and support self-determination, self-reliance, and informed self-care
d. Encourage the family to identify goals and develop a plan for achieving these goals
e. Link families and individuals with appropriate community resources
f. Follow clients to monitor outcomes and evaluate the resolution of health issues
g. Collaborate with local clinics, hospitals, and social service agencies
h. Promote accountability of health service providers for improving accessibility and acceptability of services to immigrants
i. Maintain and expand social networks

PROGRAM STRATEGIES

Registered Nurse/Community Health Advocate Team. The RN/CHA team has long been considered a core component of PHCUC strategies for bringing health education and promotion to urban communities. The RN/CHA team was selected to develop and implement a plan for fulfilling the CDPH objectives. The staff included a part-time community health nurse and full-time CHAs who are residents of the community where they work. The community health nurse works closely with CHAs in identifying prevailing health problems; an effective approach because CHAs from the neighborhood have an understanding of community health needs (Chamberlain, 1987). In addition, the nurse provides health information and promotes healthy behaviors, as well as provides ongoing health education and supervision of CHAs.

Ideally, CHAs reside in the community where they work and share the same language and socio-cultural life experiences as the people they serve. As a member of the community, the CHA is aware of community concerns, sensitive to personal issues, and comfortable in the surroundings. "Overall the CHA role is one of a bridge between the community and the formal health and social service system, an informed source of consumer health information and a person skilled in supporting and empowering community residents to increase self-reliance and control over their health." (Community Health Advocacy Training Manual, 1990, p. 2). The CHA provides an important network of support for health professionals in areas of outreach, health promotion, and health education (NINR, 1995). A nurse and health advocate team is more effective than either working alone in fostering community participation (Boema, 1987).

From the onset of the project, the staff believed that a PHC approach would be more effective when combined with case management, particularly for groups of people who are isolated and have weak ties to community. Case management as a PHC strategy may seem an unlikely choice since the term "management" implies giving up one's individual choice and self-determination. However, though other more acceptable labels, such as health advocacy, resource management, or service coordination may be applied, these activities are not necessarily synonymous. In a PHC approach, case management includes all of these activities and more. Case management as conceived in the UIC/SLIAG program is a combination of services that are planned, coordinated, and facilitated to provide an individual or family with access to services, information on programs and health services, and follow-up.

Immigrant families are often isolated within the community, not only from the systems of health and other services, but also from each other. Community-level programs are seriously challenged in reaching these groups because of economic, cultural, and linguistic barriers. Considering the barriers to care that urban immigrants face, the complex nature of their health needs, and the fragmentation of health services, case management appeared to be the most effective strategy for the project.

The strength of the case management intervention lies in the freedom to choose the best service plan from among all available services without constraint (Applebaum & Austin, 1990). The UIC/SLIAG case management project is an independent program at the local level. Though housed in a highly visible, local, family health clinic that provides bilingual and bicultural programs, the project has retained considerable autonomy.

Traditional case management is client focused; its main concern is to link clients to existing community-based services and to monitor outcomes. A PHC model for case management is more holistic, seeking to empower both the client and the community system. Clients are provided with information, health education, and skills necessary to promote self-care and self-reliance. Within the service system, the RN/CHA team provides feedback to agencies about the family, individual, and community needs promoting the development of new services or additional service capacity. As shown in Figure 1, the flow between the family and community system may be increased through PHC case management activities.

Community Well-Being

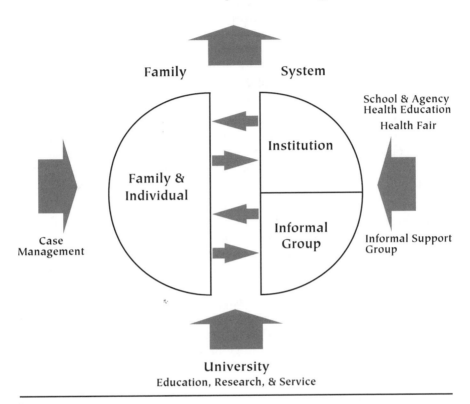

FIGURE 1.
Conceptual Diagram of PHC/SLIAG Program Implementation

The purpose of this approach is twofold: Isolated families are exposed to the diverse resources offered by the community and "glued" into the system where they can participate as service recipients. In the beginning, the RN/CHA team reflects their concerns back to the agency, but in time, with improved skills, greater knowledge, and more self-confidence, clients develop their own voices. As flow between immigrant families, local organizations, and community agencies increases, strong ties between families and the community systems are established, thus enhancing the effectiveness of the program. Ultimately these strong ties encourage mobilization of potential community resources.

Interagency Coordination. A limitation of health-service availability in the community can be resolved by increasing interagency coordination among service providers without physical capacity increases (Schermerhorn, 1976). By increasing interagency coordination, the case management program has improved access to health and social services. For example, the UIC/SLIAG project coordinates community health fairs by mobilizing local health and social service providers to increase awareness of health issues and to inform the community about what health services are available. The health fair is a cost-effective way to provide health screening, preventive healthcare services, and education to community residents in a neighborhood setting that is easily accessible and familiar (Malott, 1996). Through health fairs, isolated individuals and families become aware of available resources in the community, and local agencies have an opportunity to reach those most at risk.

Immigrant Support Groups. Immigrant support groups are another effective means of promoting health education. Enhanced family networks and social support are benefits realized by families involved with immigrant support groups. The first immigrant support group was designed to provide an opportunity for isolated families living in the same neighborhoods to meet, share experiences, and problem solve together.

Volunteers. Volunteers played a key role in health education and promotion. Clients and others in the neighborhood were offered an opportunity to become volunteers. These individuals were trained to answer the telephone, monitor clients, and provide general information on local resources and special health-related events. The experience and knowledge volunteers gained often led to employment at one of the agencies or clinics affiliated with the project. In addition, volunteers become more effective in resolving health-related problems with their neighbors. Developing a corps of volunteers is a strategy that promotes sustainability of the program. Even after the program's termination, these trained volunteers remained as a health resource, able to provide information and link families with community health services.

University Link. The role of the university in the UIC/SLIAG project has been one of not only education and service, but research. The project has provided opportunities for graduate students to conduct research on different aspects of the program. As a result of this process students have participated as observers and evaluators. The research that was generated yielded valuable information and ideas that helped program stakeholders better understand how to apply PHC principles to improve the effectiveness of the program (Keeny et al., 1993; Barron, 1994; and Buck, 1994).

Overall, the program has aspects that focus on horizontal and vertical systems. The strategic vertical system depicted in Figure 1 focuses attention on the complicated immigrant community situation where integrated comprehensive approaches are more likely to maximize program effectiveness. The combination of family/individual-level interventions within the system-level interventions provide a synergistic effect at each level. This combination of multiple levels and activities increases the chance of effective program outcomes (Weiss, 1995).

CLIENT SERVICE PLAN

Families are eligible for case management if they have health or social service needs that the PHC case management team can address. Case finding is accomplished through several sources: agency referral, outreach, self-referral, and client's referral. However, assertive outreach is the preferred mode of case finding because it provides program information at places where immigrants are likely to gather: adult education centers, churches, day-care centers, and community centers.

The family and individual assessment is divided into two parts: initial encounter and follow-up risk assessment. These assessments are a unique part of a PHC approach to case management.

Initial Encounter. The purpose of the first visit is to explain the program to the client and establish rapport. The first client encounter may take place anywhere in the community: adult educational center, church, laundromat, home, school, community centers, health fair, or over the phone. The initial contact provides an opportunity for the client to explain the family's situation, what they would like help with, and how they prioritize their needs. The CHA asks general questions concerning the family's health status and obtains demographic information. If the client is open to a second visit, an appointment is scheduled. Between the first and second visit, the CHA begins to make referrals such as appointments for primary care, prenatal care, public aid, or perhaps identifying sources of food and clothing.

Risk Assessment and Planning. The second visit is ideally in the client's home and includes a comprehensive assessment of the family's health, social support, environment, employment status, and problem-solving skills. The family is encouraged to define its own needs, set goals and priorities, and participate in planning. The plan includes steps to ensure that the client is able to access the resources they desire. Responsibility for realizing the plan is shared by family members and the case management team. During home visits, a folder with health education materials is given to the family members. Based on the goals of the plan and health needs, education is provided. At the same time, goal-related tasks are assigned to individual family members, the nurse, or CHA depending upon their skills and capacities. The service plan helps the client gain skills and knowledge about health and social services rather than automatically receiving such services.

Service Arrangements. Clients are given information about available medical and social service providers in the community and are encouraged to express their preferences. Appointments are made in the presence of the client to model self-care behavior. Arrangements are made for transportation to and from appointments if they are needed. The CHA may transport or accompany family members initially to teach them the route. If language barriers exist, the CHA may act as an interpreter and/or advocate. Clients are encouraged to make their own follow-up appointments. The CHA often advocates for clients with public aid or legal problems by interpreting forms and facilitating communication with service providers.

Monitoring. There is ongoing contact between the case management team and families to ensure that services are being provided in accordance with the plan and the desired outcomes are achieved. This follow-up is challenging as there are many families without telephones. Home visits provide an opportunity for ongoing monitoring of the family's progress and enable the team to determine if the plan has been successfully implemented and when a case can be closed.

Reassessment. Clients with complex problems usually remain in contact with the case management team until problems are resolved. However, at intervals of two to three months, all clients are re-contacted to assess changes in status and progress toward goals.

Program Evaluation. Evaluation of program activities measures intensity, breadth of service, duration, and caseload. A detailed process analysis was developed to increase the efficiency of the program implementation and the effectiveness of the program's outcomes by evaluating the combination of clients and service provider's characteristics, type, and amount of intervention. Outcome evaluation measures include the referral success rate, goal achievement rate, and self-sufficiency rate. Additional evaluation of the effects of the case management model used descriptive statistics.

IMPACT

Families and Individuals. The total number of families encountered during 1997–98 was 89, smaller than the 1995–96 number of 114. The total number of individuals was 235 (male: 99; female: 136). Of the total individuals, 226 (96%) were Hispanic and 88% were Mexican. The average age of the clients was 24 years old. Only 2% of the total individuals served were 65 or older.

Families were referred from more than ten major local agencies and organizations. In 1996–97, more than half (70 out of 89) of the families were encountered through outreach. The agency-based referrals during 1997 were only three. Agency-based referrals decreased because UIC/SLIAG staff fostered interagency networking. As a result of this collaboration, agencies in the community could make referrals to other service providers. In 1996–97, active outreach activities resulted in an increased number of non-agency-based referrals and a decline in agency-based referrals. A significant number of families were referred by clients already participating in the program.

Each client received at least one personal visit, and the number and intensity of contacts depended upon need. The maximum number of activities a family received during 1996–97 was 49 (95 hours), and the overall average time per each contact was 2 hours. Total time spent with clients during the 1996–97 year period was 1,498 hours. This is approximately 6 hours a day, excluding holidays and weekends, which means 78% of project time was devoted to case management.

The total number of activities was 876 with 33% of them classified as social services and 67% as health services. Ten percent of the total families (N = 15) spent 38% of the total time allocated for client services. One exceptional client required 90 CHA hours for 47 different activities. This extremely skewed pattern of time allocation was the result of careful investigation of the client's available resources when developing the care plan. When a family lacks available resources and has multiple problems, the resources (program time) allocated to them increases. When a family has self-help resources, such as other family members or neighbors, the program time and resources allocated to the family decreases. Education and training increases the client's available resources. Thus the care plan is monitored and managed to enhance overall program efficiency.

A total of 876 service referrals were documented in 1996–97, with an average of 4.8 referrals per client. A total of 587 referrals were made for medical service. Often, verbal agreements are used to link clients with local clinics, and several local organizations and agencies collaborated with us in providing services.

Families in this program demonstrated improved social skills, self-esteem, health behavior, knowledge, and increased use of preventive health and social services. Reducing barriers to accessing community resources has contributed to the long-term health and overall well-being of those in the program. Clients reported that barriers to access were reduced significantly by the activities of the program. These activities included assistance with transportation, accompanying the client, interpreting and translating, advocacy, information about local resources and how to use them, and education in areas of health and self-care.

In 1996, the program outcome evaluation questionnaire was adapted by the CHAs and project staff to measure the significance of the program's intervention. One of the variables the questionnaire measured was barriers to accessing health and social services. Averages of total access barrier scores from clients (N = 33) and nonclients (N = 31) were compared. Results of the two group t-test ($t = 2.44$, $p = 0.018$) were significant enough to reject the null hypothesis that the two groups were no different from each other. Results suggest that the program contributed to a reduction of client's perceived barriers in access to health and social services either directly or indirectly, thereby increasing use of health and other services by program clients as compared with nonclients. Clients of the PHC case management team had greater completion rates for referrals than clients referred by traditional referral or brokerage methods.

Local Clinics and Agencies. The program had a significant impact on local clinics. In clinics that charge on a sliding scale, long waits for appointments and services are common problems. Many clinics are operating at greater than their service capacity. Although the program's policy is to refer clients to resources in the neighborhood, the case management team realized it needed to look outside the community to ensure access to health service providers. The criteria for linking a client with alternative health or service resources include accessibility by public transportation, safety, and acceptability of services. By referring clients to resources in other neighborhoods, the program reduced the heavy burden on local clinics and increased utilization of other facilities. For instance, a clinic in a neighboring community that served an African-American population was not fully utilized until the case management team negotiated with its director to provide care for Latino clients who were underserved in their own community. Five years later, one third of the clinic's clientele is Latino and bilingual staff and primary care providers have been hired to serve them. By adding this clinic to the case management referral list, the burden on neighborhood clinics operating above the service capacity has been decreased and access improved to medical and prenatal care.

Community. The program team brought health education and resource information in Spanish to many immigrant residents, groups, and organizations. Presentations by the team raised awareness of local health problems. Other approaches were also considered when assessing the impact of the program on community health.

From an economic perspective, one method of measuring the impact of the UIC/SLIAG project is to assess its social value to the community. The social value of the program is the monetary amount contributed to the target community from the implementation of the program. In a sample of selected clients, the total value of the program was estimated using a Contingency Valuation Methods whereby the client's perceived value of the program was elicited (Park, 1997). In essence, people who had used the services (N = 63, 1994 to 1996) were asked what they were willing to pay for the service. The total value was estimated at $28,925. This amount represents the benefit (social value) of the program to the target community.

The social desirability of a program can be evaluated in terms of the cost and benefit of the program. The overall feasibility of the program can also be justified as long as the benefit exceeds the program cost. The benefit of the program exceeded the program cost. Therefore it could be concluded that this program was socially desirable and feasible to continue. Theoretically, the estimated benefit figures for the program can be an indicator of the extent of program sustainability. As long as the people served truly reported their preferences, it could be projected that they could contribute that amount of money to sustain the program.

CONCLUSION

The UIC/SLIAG program is a good demonstration of the applicability of PHC concepts to vulnerable populations in urban communities. A PHC approach combined with a case management strategy proved effective in bridging the cultural gap between the community's healthcare system and its Latino immigrant population. Findings from five years of experience verify the effectiveness of the PHC model; a model that can be applied to other communities with vulnerable populations that are isolated from existing service-delivery systems. The approach of the UIC/SLIAG program is unique among case management programs because it emphasizes the dynamic relationship between a community and its families. In this regard it expands the perspective of PHC and opens a door to new possibilities for improving the overall effectiveness of health- and social-service delivery in urban communities.

REFERENCES

Applebaum, R., & Austin, C. D. (1990). *Long-term case management: Design and evaluation*. New York: Springer-Verlag.

Barron, M. K. (1994). *Evaluation of a nurse-health advocate program for Hispanic immigrants: A primary health care intervention*. Unpublished master's project, University of Illinois at Chicago College of Nursing.

Boerma, T. (1987). The viability of the concept of a primary healthcare team in developing countries. *Social Science Medicine, 25*(6), 747–752.

Buck, K. (1994). *Women's empowerment through PHC case management*. Unpublished master's project, University of Illinois at Chicago College of Nursing.

Chamberlain, M., & Beekingham, A. (1987). Primary health care in Canada: In praise of the nurse? *International Nursing Review, 34*(6), 292–294.

Community Health Advocacy Training Manual (1990). Primary Health Care in Urban Communities Project. University of Illinois at Chicago College of Nursing.

Keeny, G., Norr, K., Swider, S., & Martinez, C. (1993). *Access to health care: Barriers among an urban Hispanic immigrant community*. Unpublished manuscript. University of Illinois at Chicago College of Nursing.

Malott, A. B. (1996). *An evaluation of a school health fair based on the concept of primary health care*. Unpublished master's thesis, University of Illinois at Chicago College of Nursing.

NINR. (1995). *Community-based health care: Nursing strategies*. Report of an NINR Priority Expert Panel, NIH Publication No. 95-3917, NIH, MD.

Park, C. G. (1997). *Economic value of nurse/community health advocate team in Hispanic communities in Chicago*. Paper available from University of Illinois at Chicago College of Nursing PHC Center.

Schermerhorn, J. (1976). Openness to interorganizational cooperation: a study of hospital managers. *Academy of Management Journal, 19*(2), 225–236.

Weiss, C. (1995). Nothing as practical as good theory: Exploring theory-based evaluation for comprehensive community initiatives for children and families. In J. P. Connell, A. C. Kubisch, L. B. Schorr, & C. H. Weiss, *New approaches to evaluating community initiatives: Concepts, methods, and context*, 65–92. Washington, DC: The Aspen Institute.

Chapter 8

Literacy for Health: Improving Health Literacy in the Inner City

BEVERLY J. MCELMURRY
MAUREEN MEEHAN
AARON G. BUSEH

Project design and implementation:
Beverly J. McElmurry, principal investigator; Stanley Diamond, co-investigator and project director; Dorothy Murphy, nurse; Willamette Douglas, community health advocate; Timothy Shanahan, director, Center for Literacy; Maureen Meehan, literacy specialist; Kathleen Tajeu, evaluation consultant.

Critical review of dissemination manuscript and drafts:
Randy Spreen Parker; Cynthia Tyska; Stanley Diamond; Dorothy Murphy; Willamette Douglas, community health advocate.

Date of project: October 1, 1992 through September 30, 1993.

This project was partially funded by a grant from the W. K. Kellogg Foundation, the National Institute for Literacy, the Lloyd A. Fry Foundation, and the University of Illinois at Chicago (UIC) College of Nursing and Center for Literacy.

HEALTH AND LITERACY
IN THE INNER CITY

Introduction

Recent studies indicate approximately one-fourth of the adults in the United States (over forty million people) had exceptionally limited literacy skills (Kirsch et al., 1993) and could be described as functionally illiterate (Wagner, 1997). These adults demonstrated literacy proficiency within the lowest of five measured levels on the 1993 National Adult Literacy Survey. While some could perform simple, routine tasks, others were unable to respond to any of the survey items. This suggests literacy is a growing concern, even in industrialized nations like the United States.

In response to these sobering statistics and based on the established correlation between health and literacy (Weiss et al., 1992; Jackson et al., 1991; and Weiss, Hart, & Pust, 1991), the Literacy for Primary Health Care (LPHC) program was developed to increase literacy skills and the effective use of these skills within a health context. Using an interdisciplinary approach, the project emphasized the participation of the learners in the curriculum development process, the use and interpretation of meaningful written materials dealing with health, and the relationship between the health literacy materials and the participants' experiences and needs. The LPHC program targeted the educational and health needs of an underserved African-American population in an inner city. Specifically, the program provided health education for selected groups of teens and young adults in one of Chicago's most economically disadvantaged communities.

This chapter illustrates a program that links health literacy with community and health development. The purpose of the project was to develop a curriculum that fosters health literacy skills and assists participants to improve their health practices. The LPHC program is also an example of collaboration between health professionals and literacy educators.

Scope of the Problem

The association between literacy and health in developing countries has been well documented (Esrey & Habicht, 1988; Coreil & Gencee, 1988; and Flegg, 1982). In many of the developing countries where literacy programs have been implemented, investigators have reported a dramatic improvement in health status indicators (Caldwell, 1979; Flegg, 1982; and Grosse & Auffrey, 1989). Although literacy was rarely measured directly in these studies, there was a strong correlation between educational attainment (a literacy proxy) and health as reflected in life expectancy, infant and child mortality, and maternal mortality rates (Epstein, 1982; Flegg, 1982; Ware, 1984; and Grosse, 1980).

In assessing this relationship between health and literacy, Grosse (1980) and Cleland and Ginneken (1988) indicated that independent of other economic factors, adult literacy, specifically the mother's literacy, had a profound effect on a child's life expectancy. Educated mothers appeared to make better use of health services, were willing to adopt new innovations, and had greater knowledge regarding health promotion and maintenance. The evidence is strong that as educational attainment rises in the nonindustrialized nations, so too do key health indicators.

In an industrialized nation like the United States, this relationship between economic development and health is even more complex. One hypothesis is that limited literacy skills often create obstacles for the development of positive self-images, employment mobility, and full participation in civic and community health activities. Despite the push for literacy programs in the United States, there are still a large number of persons whose skills do not enable them to participate fully as literate members of our society. Hence, poor comprehension of written information can affect health outcomes (Weiss, Hart, & Pust, 1991).

Approaches to Health Literacy

Often, health education programs emphasize two perspectives, literacy-free health education and revision of health materials to be more accessible to those with low literacy skills. These two perspectives will be presented here followed by a third approach, the LPHC program for the inner-city resident.

In the literacy-free training approach, health educators rely on nonwritten forms of information exchange by focusing on oral communication or the use of audio recordings, videotapes, illustrations, and demonstrations (Doak & Doak, 1985). Similarly, television remains an effective literacy-free medium for health education as well as health promotion messages. However, the specific benefits of using print cannot be ignored. Patients may leave a clinic with different degrees of comprehension after talking with a doctor or health educator, watching a demonstration, or even participating in a simulation. In general, when emphasis is placed on substituting written materials with oral, audio, and visual presentations, little attention is paid to improving the competency of those who have difficulty making sense of printed health information.

For example, mass media, including television or radio, play an important role in the dissemination of health information, but individuals still cannot, at will, refer back to thirty-second TV or radio messages. However, if the patient also has access to reinforcing print materials, full integration of new knowledge or changes in health-related behaviors can be enhanced.

The second approach focuses on revising health materials. Many agree that consumer and patient health information should be simplified. Patient and health education literature identifies a wide discrepancy between the reading comprehension of the average health consumer and the reading ability needed to understand most patient education literature (Davis et al., 1990). Simplifying written materials recognizes the value of printed health literature but raises concerns about the readability of these materials (Davis et al., 1990; Doak & Doak, 1985; Powers, 1988; Davis et al., 1996; Jackson et al., 1991; and Davis et al., 1994).

Likewise, research suggests that a significant reading gap exists between the skills of many patients and typical written health information. For example, Davis and colleagues determined the mean reading levels for patients ranged from fifth grade in a community clinic to nearly eleventh grade for patients of a private clinic. However, most of the patient education material was written at an eleventh to fourteenth grade level. University clinic informed-consent forms were at a thirteenth grade level and beyond. Moreover, the letters patients received from their physicians were written at a sixteenth to seventeenth grade level while local health-related newspaper articles were at or above an eleventh grade level (Davis et al., 1990).

Although the data were alarming, interpreting such results is partially dependent on understanding the testing and readability formulas used to assess print materials. Assigning a grade-level reading score to an adult (or a child) can be misleading. An assigned reading level score is based on the mean performance of the norm group. A score of 6.0 means that 50 percent of sixth graders in the norm group scored above this level and 50 percent scored below. There is nothing absolute about a 6.0 that suggests all sixth graders should be expected to read at this level. By definition, 50 percent will test below 6.0. The issue becomes more complex when one tries to fit an adult's reading performance into an interpretive framework designed for children. It is erroneous to assume that an adult who tests at a 6.0 level has the equivalent reading skills of an eleven-year-old child. Their skills as measured by performance on a standardized reading test may be similar, but an adult has a wealth of experience, including reading experiences, that are well beyond that of a child.

Assuming that adult reading skill levels can be identified appropriately, the second component of the readability approach is to develop printed materials to match the adult's skills. Typically this is accomplished by using formulas to evaluate various health materials. Again, caution is urged. The available computer readability programs are valuable tools but have limitations. They basically compare written material to previously analyzed criterion passages. Most formulas were developed for use within standard educational settings and the criterion passages were generally drawn from this setting as well. The formulas analyze semantic and syntactic features and, based on a comparison with the criterion passages, assign a grade level. Most formulas predict readability based on some combination of the following factors: average sentence length, percentage of words not on a list of frequently used words, syllable counts, and numbers of sentences.

Perhaps the greatest threat to the validity of formula predictions is the use of technical terms and jargon throughout written healthcare materials. Formulas which incorporate lists of frequently used words will elevate readability of these materials because of technical vocabulary. Medical terms are often multisyllabic, another factor that will elevate the readability score, and readability is most likely further inflated simply because these terms are repeated. The formulas cannot account for the fact that adults may be very familiar with such terms, therefore the use of these terms may not limit comprehension. For instance, diabetics are familiar with the term "insulin," transplant patients know about "anti-rejection," cancer patients are all too familiar with "chemotherapy" and "radiation." While these terms would not necessarily affect comprehension, they would definitely elevate readability predictions.

Readability formulas are also limited in that they do not address the critical aspects of content, format, or organizational features which are known to contribute to the comprehensibility of the text. The formulas are not designed to consider motivation or prior knowledge as contributing factors. It is the interaction among all these variables that makes the study of readability so complex, and the use of only readability formulas too simplistic. A real danger of applying readability formulas to health education is the abuse of formulas within the writing process. If an author creates health information material and then runs a computer readability formula, he/she may decide to make revisions that will supposedly improve readability. However, this "write-run formula-revise-run formula" method of creating health education materials can actually result in less accessible text. Text readability scores will improve based on word choice and sentence structure. Yet, substituting the meaningful health word with other terms or shortening sentences can actually decrease comprehension (Pearson & Campbell, 1981). Minimizing technical language may decrease comprehensibility. The formulas cannot account for a target population who may be highly motivated or have extensive prior knowledge when facing critical health conditions, factors that may make material more understandable in spite of higher readability scores.

The LPHC project set out to improve both the health and literacy competency of inner-city residents. The definition of health literacy used in the project emphasized the ability of the participants to comprehend written and printed health information, the skills to use health information in their lives, and the development of values and attitudes that support a healthy lifestyle. While recognizing the benefits and limitations of delivering literacy-free health education programs or revising health-related materials to make the content more accessible, the LPHC approach addressed literacy skill development within a context of health promotion.

Through a unique collaboration between adult literacy specialists and primary health care providers, LPHC developed a training curriculum based on a different definition of health literacy. While most nursing education programs include some content on the importance of considering the literacy level of health education recipients, the amount of instruction on this topic varies. Likewise, the international literature on health education does not directly address the ability of lay community health workers to assess the literacy levels of the people with whom they work. In this application, the primary objective was to develop the literacy skills needed to use and interpret written health information. To achieve this goal, the LPHC curriculum was developed to support the nurse/health advocate team's assessment of the community's health education needs. The curriculum is a tool to complement the expertise of the health education team and to more effectively deliver community-based health education for those with a wide range of literacy skills.

Design and Implementation of the LPHC Curriculum

The principles of PHC were used to implement the LPHC program. A public health nurse and a community health advocate worked for five years in efforts to improve health outcomes in a community that was 98 percent African American with more than 50% percent living below the poverty level. This team successfully addressed a wide range of health concerns for members of this community who were committed to making a difference for their families. In spite of the community's acceptance of traditional health education methods (single topic, single session presentations), the team wanted an opportunity to better evaluate the transfer of learning and actual skill application in daily activities, that is, the changes in health behavior.

The application of PHC concepts in the LPHC project incorporated certain fundamental values common to the overall process of development in the target community, but with emphasis on their application in the field of health. As a concept, PHC emphasizes that health is an integral component of development even within urban settings. Health is influenced by social, cultural, economic, biological, and environmental factors as well as the individual's literacy level. The LPHC project created an opportunity for individuals to achieve better health by involving them in actions to access resources and thus develop greater self-sufficiency and self-care. Modeling a health curriculum on literacy education required the involvement of participants in the education process and encouraged engagement with reading and writing tasks related to self-sufficiency and self-care. Incorporating literacy development into a health education program meant fully integrating reading and writing in a way that ensures individuals gain health knowledge. To succeed, the curriculum development was dependent on the expertise of the health educators to assure appropriate content and on the literacy educators to assure specific reading and writing skill development.

From a PHC perspective, the selection of content was guided by at least two considerations: What had the nurse/advocate team learned about this urban population after working with them for several years; and what had community members indicated were essential health areas about which they should be knowledgeable or literate. The combination of health and literacy expertise led ultimately to an education and training program with health education objectives and related literacy skill development for each unit. Although knowledge transfer was important, the long-term use of new knowledge was the ultimate goal.

Given the past PHC initiatives in the target community, the experiences of the project team, and input from community-based organizations, young parents were identified as a population seeking ways to maintain and improve their health and that of their children. Hence, young parents became the target population for the LPHC program.

The entire curriculum comprised seven units (Table 1) and was designed to be taught by a nurse and a CHA over a twelve-week period (two hours per session; four hours per week). The curriculum was refined after each successive

TABLE 1.
Health Literacy Teaching Modules

Introduction of the Program

Perspectives on Nutrition

Human Development

Parenting Skills: Effective Discipline and Guidance

Family Violence: Prevention, Strategies, Alternatives

Human Sexuality: Family Planning, HIV/AIDS, and Other STDs

Safety/CPR: Creating a Safe Home Environment

Full curriculum is available from ERIC Documents #404436.

implementation and also was adapted for the skills and interests of learners in each instructional group.

Four community organizations participated in the literacy for health program. One group of participants included nearly sixty parents whose children had been removed by the state's child welfare agency due to abuse, neglect, or endangerment. Another group of parents were from the Parent Education Center in a public housing unit. A third group that enrolled were young pregnant women and new mothers living in a small residential facility that provided them shelter, counseling, and education services. The final group included students at an alternative high school in the community. Participants from the schools were young parents or had substantial child-care responsibilities for younger siblings. In spite of the original target audience of young, single mothers, the parent participants' ages ranged from young teens to early thirties and at one site included both mothers and fathers. The age range of parents was not an issue; however, including fathers in one group led the team to conclude that a separate father's group might be more effective.

TEACHING STRATEGIES

The LPHC program used a participatory framework, a critical tenant of the PHC model. In this program, decision making was shared among the learners and staff. The participants' knowledge, skills, and experiences were valued and respected and provided the foundation upon which learning activities were built. This participatory process created a climate of acceptance that fostered the acquisition of skills and knowledge related to the health literacy curriculum.

Initially, a public health nurse and the CHA delivered training with input and support from the adult literacy specialist. These health educators met weekly with the university-based literacy specialist and project coordinator to review the outcomes of lessons and to plan for upcoming sessions. Developing a sequential, integrated health curriculum that included multiple sessions per topic and focused on assessing behavioral outcomes was a new experience for the health educators. These educators taught nutrition concepts and the related reading-writing skills in class and followed up with field trips and assignments to foster experiential learning. For example, the project included trips to the Museum of Science and Industry to look at nutrition displays and interact with computer software related to nutrition. This was followed by trips to the grocery story to encourage practical application of these nutrition concepts. Students also organized class parties to demonstrate new ways of food preparation that reflected changed cooking habits.

As the program progressed, more active involvement of the adult literacy instructor was necessary to fully integrate reading and writing strategies. At later stages in the implementation of the curriculum, the CHA assumed a stronger teaching role. Eventually, the CHA and the literacy teacher became the teaching team with technical support from the public health nurse. It was critically important that both a health educator and literacy specialist compose this unique teaching team to insure the integration of health and literacy content.

While trained health advocates can deliver acceptable and cost-effective programs in the community, they will always need the support and expertise of a literacy specialist and public health nurse when working with groups who have limited literacy and real health threats. For example, journal writing is a literacy enhancement activity, but when read by a health specialist, it often reveals health issues not fully understood by the writer, a literacy teacher, or lay health advocate.

MATERIALS

Neither standard health education nor literacy education materials were used exclusively. Health-related materials were selected based upon what the participants encountered in the course of their everyday activity. Health education topics suggested materials for a health literacy program. For example, nutrition materials included food labels, money-saving coupons, food advertisements, menus, recipes, and nutrition charts. Vaccination schedules, medicinal packaging, and forms for obtaining healthcare services were filled with important health education content and served as a rich source of reading and writing activities.

Learners were also encouraged to create their own materials by writing about their health experiences. Journals were used to record health-related events in the parents' lives and those of their children. This was a new opportunity for many who had never documented symptoms, maintained vaccination records, created schedules to monitor medicine intake, wrote lists of questions for doctors prior to a visit, or used calendars to schedule appointments. Dialogue journals were used to communicate with the teachers. Participants could write questions or share health concerns with the teachers, and the teachers provided written feedback responses in the journals and follow-up on an individual basis. Journal writing was also explored as a means of venting frustration or anger within the child development and discipline units. The health journal was promoted as a class activity and as a health habit that could be maintained long after the training ended.

Family health education stresses the importance of understanding the influence children have on the health habits of their parents. For example, Murphy et al. (1996) observed that children can be an impetus to promoting healthy adult eating habits. In the LPHC program intergenerational health literacy activities were designed with both the parent and the child in mind. The purpose for such activities was to increase knowledge of disease prevention, improve reading skills, and enhance parenting skills. Further exploration of family and community systems could be expected to reveal acceptable and effective health literacy materials.

EVALUATION PROCEDURES

The LPHC project was initially funded by a one-year grant from the National Institute for Literacy. Within the limits of the available funding, the team had to make decisions regarding the allocation of funds for development, implementation, and evaluation. Within these limitations, the project staff took a comprehensive approach to evaluation. The specific evaluation techniques were developed in consultation with an external evaluator from the UIC Department of Medical Education. These evaluation procedures evolved over the course of the project and were a result of the team's collaborative reflection on the implementation process. The available funding permitted this quarter-time external evaluator to work with the team for the first six months. The concentration of funds on development and implementation was appropriate, yet it would have been useful to have an external evaluator for the full project period.

The Comprehensive Adult Student Assessment System (CASAS) Health Care Materials Appraisal Form was selected as an initial screening to obtain information on general skill levels. This instrument, like all CASAS assessments, was designed for adults and had particularly high face validity given the health literacy focus of the project. The CASAS does not yield grade-level scores which may easily be misinterpreted when applied to adults. Based on test performance, participants are assigned a literacy level. Levels range from A which is the lowest level (those who are unable to effectively use print materials) to the highest level D (equivalent to a high school entry level or above). The wide range of literacy skills among the participants was apparent: 0% in Level A; 23% in Level B; 28% in Level C; and 49% in Level D. This screening alerted teachers to participants who might have significant difficulty during the program or who may have more highly developed literacy skills and need to be challenged during the course. The instructors observed that a few participants actively avoided this screening. It was later concluded based on the instructors' subsequent experiences and observations that these participants would most likely have scored in the lower levels.

The CASAS served as an effective screening instrument. However, given the number of contact hours and the health-specific goals of the program, it was not appropriate to focus the evaluation on measuring significant reading gains through typical pre- and post-test literacy assessment procedures.

A number of formative evaluation methods were implemented throughout the project to evaluate the process of learning, changes in literacy, the relevancy of the content, and increases in health knowledge. These methods were used by the teachers on an ongoing basis to better understand the effects of training. Questions asked throughout the program included: What was going on in the classroom? How were students using the health information? What was the relevancy of the class and the curriculum to the life of the participants? What could the teachers do to make the curriculum more meaningful? Specific LPHC evaluation activities included:

- A pre-/post-questionnaire about health attitudes and habits as well as reading practices. These questionnaires, along with individual portfolios containing samples of participants' work, were used to evaluate knowledge, interest, and concerns regarding health, as well as changes in health-related behavior and practices.
- Practicums were used to evaluate how participants applied the classroom learning to real-world situations. For example, a visit to a supermarket assessed in practical terms how students applied lessons on nutrition. A visit to a clinic evaluated skills in accessing the healthcare system. A lesson on HIV/AIDS went well beyond content knowledge when participants went out into their community to identify clinics, hospitals, and hospice facilities that serve AIDS patients or provide testing.
- Observations by researchers and instructors were used to assess the level of interaction between participants and teachers as well as among participants themselves. As the health educators moved away from the traditional deficit learning model (the teacher has the content and must give it to the learner), they noticed an increase in involvement and interaction among participants.
- Instructors maintained journals in which they reflected upon the training. These were used during staff meetings to consider changes in their teaching strategies or lesson modifications.
- Instructors routinely held informal conferences with participants before, during, and after class. Such contacts were frequently initiated by the participants and provided an opportunity for the instructors to further evaluate the effectiveness of the teaching and whether the health literacy curriculum was relevant to participants' lives.
- Final evaluation interviews were conducted with individuals and groups of participants.

In choosing to work with community agencies, the project staff adapted to the schedules of the participants which meant it was not always possible to provide participants from different agencies the same number of instructional hours. Based on the available instructional hours at each site, the instructors tailored the curriculum to be responsive to the needs of the learners.

CHALLENGES

The project staff recognized that they were constructing a curriculum that differed from traditional health or literacy education programs. Although the end product was improved by incorporating the expertise of both disciplines, this type of collaboration is time intensive. Curriculum revisions based on preliminary field testing proved inadequate. It was necessary for the team to review units after each teaching experience to achieve the desired balance between both health and literacy goals.

The nurse/health advocate teaching team contributed a level of health knowledge beyond that of a literacy teacher. However, they were not initially comfortable with the ongoing modifications needed to address the needs of learners with wide ranging literacy skills. They grew to appreciate the additional demands of developing and teaching an ongoing, sequential program as opposed to the traditional single-topic presentation. The merger between health and literacy required the health education instructors to develop new ways of teaching, and the literacy instructor to value the content expertise of the health educator.

LESSONS LEARNED

1. Delivering an integrated curriculum or pairing a literacy and health educator as a teaching team requires support and extensive staff development. It takes time to develop a collaborative relationship between different specialists and to provide opportunities for each to learn from the other. There is a delicate balance needed to deliver lessons in a way that develops literacy skills, enhances health-content knowledge and ultimately improves health and related behaviors.

2. The original health literacy model proposed a nurse/health advocate teaching team with the nurse serving as a mentor to provide both teaching and content knowledge support to the health advocate. The health advocate was to assume greater teaching responsibility as she gained experience. The literacy specialist was to consult on curriculum development and delivery, attend project staff meetings, and be available to do site visits to provide more definitive feedback and recommendations. While the proposed model worked well, more extensive involvement by the literacy specialist was found to be beneficial. To provide more timely training and to model effective literacy teaching strategies, a literacy teacher was added to the actual teaching team. At that point, the literacy teacher and the health advocate assumed primary teaching responsibility with continued support from the nurse, adult literacy program specialist, and project personnel.

3. Health education touches critically important aspects of participants' lives, and teachers need to assume multiple roles in order to both serve the participants and achieve the program's health goals. An LPHC goal might be to develop the literacy skills and health knowledge necessary for a woman to access appropriate resources should she become involved in an

abusive relationship. However, when a program participant comes to class obviously abused and seeking help, the health professional needs to respond immediately. Participants in crisis cannot wait for a training program to develop the skills needed to avoid or respond to such situations. This forces the health professional into a case manager's role. This proved very frustrating to the health educators who felt pulled between the goals of the LPHC project and the immediate needs of the participants. Considerable time had to be devoted to helping resolve participants' personal circumstances related to such topics as domestic violence, child abuse, and sexually transmitted disease. Balancing the role of health educator versus case manager was found to be especially challenging in the target community which had limited resources and health providers.

4. Real-life circumstances often interfered with the participants' desires to learn and attend class. Literacy teachers were often challenged by learners who missed classes and had legitimate reasons for not completing activities. This often resulted in the need to modify planned lessons. For example, one nutrition unit was based on the participants' recordings of their eating habits over three days prior to class. However, when only a few participants had recorded their food consumption, achievement of nutrition content goals was delayed and compromised. This is an issue that health educators do not typically need to address when teaching single-topic presentations.

5. The curriculum worked well for the intended audience (i.e., young mothers). In sites which included fathers some units proved challenging. For example, in one class there was considerable tension between participants and the instructors as well as among the participants during the Family Violence unit. The project staff decided to carefully evaluate future classes and separate them by gender, if necessary, for this topic. Thus, another alternative might be to use a male teaching team to deliver health literacy to a fathers' group.

6. LPHC has the potential to effectively communicate knowledge as well as change health attitudes and behaviors. Although the evaluation process was evolving and further testing of the curriculum was needed, the extensive interviews with participants and the final questionnaires suggested there was a positive change in attitudes and behavior. For example, after the nutrition unit participants regularly reported the involvement of family members in implementing nutritional changes while planning meals and shopping. Changes in child-rearing practices seemed to be positively influenced by the length of the program. Parents had the opportunity to observe and record their current practices or approaches to discipline, explore alternatives in class, and then go home to try new methods with the support and encouragement of the teachers and fellow participants. Parents were also supported in using reading and writing to investigate, plan, implement, and assess such changes.

7. Another major lesson learned was the benefit of the collaborative effort between the College of Nursing, College of Education, and the community.

Interdisciplinary partnerships are a significant factor to consider when implementing LPHC programs. Prior to this project, the nursing and health literacy specialists had not collaborated. Therefore, a level of trust and commonality had to be established between the two disciplines. Second, the two professions are highly autonomous and professionals from the two departments had to relinquish some independent operations to function in a spirit of collegiality. Ultimately, the project benefited from the strengths of both disciplines.

CONCLUSIONS

LPHC can serve as a model for developing effective health education programs for those with limited literacy skills. Seeking and maintaining health requires access to information to make decisions and solve problems. Parents have many questions and concerns. When are symptoms severe enough to warrant a visit to a doctor? What foods should I include or exclude from my family's diet? Where can I find out more about a health problem or concern? What are appropriate discipline techniques for children of different ages and stages of development? There are no simple answers to these questions; rather, parents need a variety of skills, including literacy skills, to effectively manage their family's health.

The LPHC project demonstrated the potential benefits of incorporating literacy into health education. If resources are not available to implement a fully integrated LPHC program, health educators would benefit from staff development on literacy teaching techniques and strategies. Likewise, the project demonstrated that literacy teachers do not have the expertise to comprehensively address health education. Adult literacy programs would benefit from establishing a partnership in which health educators have an opportunity to present health lessons within adult literacy programs and with the support of the adult literacy teachers.

REFERENCES

Caldwell, J. C. (1979). Education as a factor in mortality decline: An examination of Nigerian data. *Population Studies, 33*, 395–413.

Cleland, J. G., & Van Ginneken, J. K. (1988). Maternal education and child survival in developing countries: The search for pathways of influence. *Social Science and Medicine, 27*, 357–68.

Corcil, J. & Gencee, E. (1988). Adaptation of oral rehydration therapy among Haitian mothers. *Social Science and Medicine, 27*, 87–96.

Davis, C., Bocchini, J. A., Fredrickson, D., Arnold, C., Mayeaux, E. J., Murphy, P. W., Jackson, R. H., Hanna, N., & Peterson, M. (1996). Parent comprehension of polio vaccine information pamphlets. *Pediatrics, 97*(6), 804–538.

Davis, T. C., Crouch, M. A., Wills, G., Miller, S., & Abdehou, D. M. (1990). The gap between patient reading comprehension and the readability of patient education materials. *The Journal of Family Practice, 31*(5), 533–538.

Davis, T. C., Mayeaux, E. J., Fredrickson, D., Bocchini, J. A., Jackson, R. H., & Murphy, P. W. (1994). Reading ability of parents compared with reading level of pediatric patient education materials. *Pediatrics, 93*(3), 460–68.

Doak, C. C., & Doak, L. G. (1985). *Teaching patients with low literacy skills.* Philadelphia: Lippincott.

Epstein, T. S. (1982). The social context of education and health. *Health Policy Education, 3,* 71–90.

Esrey, S. A., & Habicht, J. P. (1988). Maternal literacy modifies the effect of toilets and piped water on infant survival in Malaysia. *American Journal of Epidemiology, 127,* 1079–87.

Flegg, A. T. (1982). Inequality of income, literacy, and medical care as determinants of infant mortality in underdeveloped countries. *Population Studies, 36,* 441–458.

Grosse, R. N. (1980). Interrelation between health and population: Observations derived from field experiences. *Social Science and Medicine, 14,* 99–120.

Grosse, R. N. & Auffrey, C. (1989). Literacy and health status in developing countries. *Ann. Review of Public Health, 10,* 281–97.

Hunter, C. S. (1985). *Adult literacy in the United States.* New York: McGraw-Hill.

Jackson, R. H., Davis, T. C., Bairnsfather, L. E., George, R., Crouch, M., & Gault, H. (1991). Patient readability: An overlooked problem in health care. *Southern Medical Journal, 84*(10), 1172–1175.

Kirsch, I. S., Jungebut, A., Jenkins, L., & Kolstad, A. (1993). *Adult literacy in America: A first look at the results of the national Adult Literacy Survey.* Princeton: Educational Testing Service.

Murphy, P. W., Davis, T. C., Mayeaux, J. E., Sentell, T., Arnold, C., & Rebouche, C. (1996). Teaching nutrition education in adult learning centers: Linking literacy, health care, and the community. *Journal of Community Health Nursing, 13*(3), 149–158.

Pearson, P. D., & Campbell, K. (1981). Comprehension of text structures. In J. T. Guthrie (Ed.), *Comprehension and teaching: Research reviews.* Newark, D. E.: International Reading Association.

Powers, R. D. (1988). Emergency department patient literacy and the readability of patient directed materials. *Annals of Emergency Medicine, 17,* 124–126.

Wagner, D. A. (1997). Series preface. In A. C. Tuijnman, I. S. Kirsch, & D. A. Wagner (Eds.), *Adult basic skills: Innovations in measurement and policy analysis.* Cresskill, NJ: Hampton Press Inc.

Ware, H. (1984). Effects of maternal education, women's roles, and child care on child mortality. *Population Development Review, 10,* 194–214.

Weiss, B. D., Hart, G., McGee, D. L., & D'Estelle, S. (1992). Health status of illiterate adults: Relation between literacy and health status among persons with low literacy skills. *Journal of American Board of Family Practice, 5*(3), 257–264.

Weiss, B. D., Hart, G., Pust, R. E. (1991). The relationship between literacy and health. *Journal of Health Care for the Poor and Underserved, 1,* 43–55.

Chapter 9

The Chicago Health Corps: Community Service as a Transformative Experience

PEG DUBLIN
TODD HISSONG

The author wishes to recognize present and former Chicago Health Corps staff:

Present

Program Co-Directors: Dr. Richard A. Wansley and Dr. Beverly J. McElmurry
Program Coordinator: Paru Shah
Team Leaders: Matthew Shullick, Cynthia McKay, Hannah Park, Karynn Cavero
Evaluation Consultant: Aaron Buseh
Office Manager: Elsa Almaguer
Communications Specialist: Todd Hissong

Past

Former Program Manager: Ada Mary Gugenheim
Former Program Coordinators: Virginia Warren, Spring Gombe, Donell Bullock
Former Team Leaders: Teresita Te, Tamika Lee, Lawrence Franowicz

We would also like to express our sincere gratitude to our funders: the Corporation for National Service, the Health Resource and Services Administration, the Chicago Community Trust, the Otho S. A. Sprague Memorial Institute, the Lloyd A. Fry Foundation, the United States Environmental Protection Agency, the Polk Bros. Foundation, and the Washington Square Health Foundation, Inc.

Chicago is a city rich in racial and ethnic diversity, architecture, and music, and has a history of involving community residents in improving the world around them through social and educational reform, community service, and neighborhood efforts to reduce violence. Chicago also has long-standing patterns of segregated housing, racial health disparities, a declining job market, and decreasing governmental support for communities and social services. A shocking 33% of Chicago's children live in poverty, approximately 42% of whom are African American, 33% white, and 25% Hispanic. Data collected over the past several years reflects a grim picture:

- In 1992, 107 babies per 1,000 born in Chicago had low birth weight, well above the statewide rate and even surpassing New York City (both 78 per 1,000).
- Approximately one in five first births are to unwed teen-aged mothers who have not completed high school.
- The majority of Chicago's citizens live in medically underserved communities (Voices for Illinois Children, 1994).

Good health provides the foundation for a child's social, emotional, intellectual, and physical development, but as traditional sources of support diminish, Chicago families are becoming increasingly isolated while their neighborhoods suffer continued deterioration.

The Chicago Health Corps is an AmeriCorps*USA program established in 1994 by the Corporation for National Service in partnership with the Health Resources and Services Administration (HRSA) and developed and administered by the Illinois Area Health Education Centers (AHEC) program and the University of Illinois at Chicago (UIC) College of Nursing. Each year 28–34 Health Corps Members are recruited into the program to serve a term of service (one year) either full- or part-time. These Members are chosen from two pools of applicants: health professions students and community residents. Health professions students may be in school and embarked on a health career, are deferring a year, are participating in the program part-time, or have completed their undergraduate degree and are considering a health professions future. Community residents considered for the program have been recommended by former Corps Members or have been referred by the program's community partners. All of the participants are selected based on their history of community service, interest in pursuing a health career, personal recommendations, and their ability to complete the program. The overall objectives of the Chicago Health Corps embrace the primary health care (PHC) framework by teaming these community residents and health professions students together to provide health service in existing community health and educational settings.

Following a two-week pre-service training, Corps Members are assigned to a community health center, social service agency, or educational setting with supervision provided by that particular site. Every effort is made to match the needs and geographic location of the site with the Corps Member's interests and residence. Corps Members provide a combination of outreach, health education, home visits, and case management services to address unmet health needs identified by the community. During the year, Corps Members receive a minimal stipend, child-care reimbursement, health insurance, and transportation assistance. At the conclusion of their term of service, Members receive an educational award which may be used for college, vocational training, or to repay student loans. Throughout the year, Members receive ongoing training in health issues, cultural competence, community awareness, accessing social services, skill building, and participate in a mentoring program which exposes them to a variety of health careers and teaches them how to pursue further education.

POPULAR EDUCATION

Two conceptual frameworks guide Chicago Health Corps training: popular education and capacity-building community development. Popular education (inspired by Brazilian educator Paulo Freire) involves people in group efforts identifying their own issues, critically analyzing the cultural, political, and socioeconomic roots of problems, and developing strategies to positively change their lives (Freire, 1973). The premise of Freire's work is that education is not neutral and is always within a social context; its priority is ordinary people taking responsibility for cooperative study and action. Freire recognizes the link between emotion and the motivation to act, the need for curriculum to be based on the life experiences of students (rather than being determined by "experts"), and the importance of dialogue between students and facilitators (Freire, 1973). The facilitator's job is to help identify issues which spark emotion in the students. Together, the student and facilitator identify the root causes of these issues and seek strategies to resolve problems (Freire, 1973).

An example of our application of popular education is in the way we train Corps Members to make health presentations in the community. We start the session by introducing the subject with a "trigger"—a projective device based on a generative theme experienced by people in the group to engage the student in the topic. For example, we might show a picture of a teacher pumping education into a student's head, similar to a car being filled with gasoline. Through a series of questions leading from the objective to the subjective, the facilitator is able to engage participants in a meaningful conversation about what's wrong with "banking education" and lead into a discussion of an alternative, more relevant educational method.

Some Corps Members have had negative educational experiences which have fostered feelings of failure. Because the method of popular education is based on lived experiences, the participants are on a level playing field, which is of critical importance in a program with such divergent educational backgrounds. The group is able to move from discussion of personal experiences with the educational system to the discovery of more relevant, meaningful dialogue that can then be applied in their service experience. The facilitator who utilizes this process needs to be nonjudgmental, able to facilitate 7emotionally charged encounters, and engage full participation of all group Members.

Popular education is used within the Health Corps to facilitate the Members' analysis of the healthcare system and public health issues such as lead poisoning in Chicago, the asthma epidemic among Chicago's school children, and low breastfeeding rates in underserved communities. This methodology encourages the development of new strategies for combating these issues and engaging full participation of both Corps Members and community residents. One of our goals is that Corps Members will begin to apply popular education in their community settings and develop a deeper understanding over the course of their lifetimes.

IMPLEMENTING PRIMARY HEALTHCARE KEY CONCEPTS

The Chicago Health Corps is divided into three issue-based teams: Environmental Health (lead poisoning prevention and asthma management for children), Youth Health Education (self-care strategies for school-age children), and Personal Health (health promotion and social support for vulnerable populations such as new mothers and seniors). Corps Members are placed in a public hospital, a youth organization, two community-based social service agencies, four public elementary schools, and seven community health centers. In all of these sites, Corps Members strive to involve individuals and communities in the planning of health-related activities. Member training stresses that health promotion is inextricably linked to social and economic development, and therefore their activities lead them to other related concerns such as housing, jobs, education, violence prevention, poverty and hunger. One service site that Corps Members were assigned to was a senior citizen high-rise in the heart of Chicago. The site supervisor described one of the more unusual, but nonetheless essential services Corps Members provided:

> They have helped us establish some links with getting people out of their apartments and back into their community. One of our Chicago Health Corps volunteers has started an art program, and the art program has engaged both men and women. We've found a gap in our services in that we have not been able to find things for the older single men to do, besides playing pool, or whatever, that some men have never done in their lives. The art program has provided them an activity to do that. . . . They have made a big, big difference.

CAPACITY BUILDING

Corps Members do not take the place of existing workers, but seek to expand the capacity of the agency. Corps Members are introduced to concepts of capacity-building (based on the work of John McKnight & John Kretzmann, 1993) which offers an alternative method of assessing communities by looking at capacities and gifts rather than deficiencies and needs. Members learn to recognize their own individual gifts and capacities, identify associations within communities, and begin the process of mobilizing community capacity. As a result, they often have the opportunity to explore and subsequently intervene to reduce barriers to accessing healthcare. These barriers may include language, transportation, child care, misinformation, and lack of trust. Corps Members routinely translate, accompany, listen, provide referrals, and problem solve in a culturally competent and sensitive manner.

One example of health education and outreach that Corps Members are involved with is the promotion of breastfeeding, which provides numerous health benefits but is rarely supported in low-income communities. Developing a relationship with a new mother around breastfeeding provides a window of opportunity to discuss other important health issues including nutrition, prenatal care, parenting, well-child care, maternal care, and available maternal-child health and social services. Additionally, since Corps Members are able to take the time to develop relationships with clients, unexpected benefits are often encountered. At one site, a Corps Member asked a pregnant teen if she was interested in learning about breastfeeding. The teen responded with a forceful "No," but changed her mind when she overheard the Corps Member talking to another expectant mother. The Corps Member then spent two hours with the teen and enrolled her in an upcoming breastfeeding class. The Corps Member explains:

> As we talked one of the topics that came up was about school; this teen who is 17 years old, had dropped out at the age of 15. When she found out how close we were in age and how I worked and went to school full-time, she asked me about going back to get her GED. I told her I would find out for her. She now calls me at least twice a week and we talk and she has agreed to go to a GED program starting next term. From this experience I think we both learned from each other. She looked at herself in a new way. And now I look at the mothers with more understanding than I ever had before.

Corps Member involvement in asthma management has provided several excellent opportunities to implement key PHC concepts. The Open Airways in Schools program is an American Lung Association curriculum designed to help asthmatic school-age children improve their knowledge and management of their condition. Corps Members are implementing this six-week program, which provides education and social support to the children, via the formation of an asthma club. In PHC terms, education, prevention, and health promotion (the curriculum) is taking place by multisectoral action (the Lung Association, the school, the Health Corps) presented by culturally competent and acceptable role models (the Corps Members). This project has the added benefit of providing Corps Members with a deepened experience in inner-city school environments.

The Environmental Health Team has been involved with a variety of health promotion and prevention efforts that maximize individual and community involvement in their planning. Following repeated exposure to high lead levels in an overcrowded elementary school located in the Little Village neighborhood, Health Corps Members (working along side the Little Village Environmental Justice project) developed a lead poisoning curriculum for the students and conducted educational lead workshops for interested parents. As a result of the health education activities, many children expressed interest in forming an Environmental Justice Club. This club (comprising students, Corps Members and the Little Village project staff) planned social and educational activities throughout the school term. At the end of the school year, Corps Members who had been working with a local Environmental Justice Coordinator decided to offer an Environmental Justice Summer Course. Thirteen students participated in this intensive summer program which met five days a week, three and a half hours a day. The children and Corps Members engaged in various activities including the completion of a toxic inventory of the school building and grounds, utilized the Internet to research hazardous materials, and took weekly field trips to environmental sites (a sustainable agriculture farm, an agricultural high school, and sites that pose a threat to the environment). Students were introduced to experiential and adventure-based education through team-building exercises. Parents became involved with these efforts as well and helped plan other related activities.

COLLABORATION

Collaboration is central to the structure and philosophy of the Chicago Health Corps and the program is made up of many partnerships. The primary partnership lies between the program co-directors: The UIC College of Nursing and the Illinois AHEC program, a statewide organization whose mission is to increase PHC capacity in underserved areas by facilitating programmatic links between health professions schools and the community. Dr. Richard Wansley, executive director of the Illinois AHEC program, describes the partnership as a perfect fit with his organization:

> The Chicago Health Corps was attractive to me and our AHEC program because it provides an intensive opportunity for people interested in health careers, before they actually begin that training to become a health professional, to spend a year or more of their time working in community settings where the communities are underserved and where there are people who truly need primary health care services.

The UIC College of Nursing is responsible for hiring and housing the staff and providing training space for the Corps Members. Because of the central role the UIC College of Nursing plays in the program, community partner agencies and community Members have an increased accessibility to university resources such as the Internet, library services, and faculty members. Corps Members who have never set foot in a university come on a regular basis for in-service training, meet with Health Corps staff, attend computer classes, learn from university faculty, and acclimate to the environment. A former Corps Member describes the change he has experienced:

> As an undergraduate, my concept of the university was almost like something sacred unto itself. It was like you had this building that nothing really needs to go in and nothing really needs to go out. So in my mind, it really goes along the line of bench work science, and something is really preserved inside. Yet, the next question you really have to ask is "Then what's the use of it? If it's all stuffed inside institutional walls, it's focusing on itself." The emphasis to use the resources of a university to involve community is really paramount to have a lot more kids understand the resources available to them. If that relationship is there, than the university becomes more real, concrete to them, and it becomes more interactive. It's the difference between, "The university came in and we worked with them," rather than "The university came in and did their study." So my concept is a lot broader. Now I'll ask a lot more of the university to work with the projects that I am working on.

As for the university's role in this partnership, Dr. Beverly J. McElmurry (professor, associate dean of the UIC College of Nursing, and co-director of the Chicago Health Corps) has this to offer:

> The major land grant institution is a public institution, is the people's institution, and therefore it should be responsive to what the people are saying are the things they want attended to, the technical resources that they want from the university.

The program management team is composed of representatives of university health professions and college institutions, local/federal health agencies, and site supervisors from community health settings where Corps Members are placed. The program management team helps to set policy and assists with long-range planning. Site supervisors meet bi-monthly and address issues of placement, supervision, training needs, and program planning.

Throughout their entire term of service, Corps Member partnerships (a health professions student matched with a community resident) provide a rich diversity of experience. Corps Members have the opportunity to get to know and work closely with people from very different backgrounds, different life and educational experiences, cultures, ages, and ethnicity. Within their teams, Corps Members exchange areas of expertise: How to conduct oneself doing door-to-door outreach, how best to instruct and demonstrate to a Latina mother proper breastfeeding positioning, how to teach ten-year-olds conflict resolution, how to devise a lead poisoning follow-up protocol for family practitioners, etc. The value of this "immersion experience" is profound. One Corps Member describes her year:

> I cannot stress enough how valuable my AmeriCorps experience has been. I only wish more Americans were able to have such an experience. Not only does it instill the value of community service, provide needed educational stipends, give experience beyond education, but most importantly the program unifies our diverse nation. The Health Corps consists of individuals from all different walks of life. We've found our common ground and are working together for a common goal. I honestly don't know of any other program that accomplishes this. I have learned the value behind the American motto, E Pluribus Unum (out of many, one).

LESSONS LEARNED

Admittedly, the Health Corps experience can create tension and conflict for Members as well as the potential for growth, and it is one of the more challenging aspects of the program for everyone involved. In one site, a Corps Member who has completed graduate level course work was raised in a suburban community and has worked in university and healthcare institutions is paired with a woman who has not completed high school, is the mother of three children, whose first language is Spanish, and has little work experience outside her home. It took months of hard work (and one conflict mediation session) for these Members to learn to work together and understand each other. Now they consider each other to be family.

For many of our Members, the program provides their first experience in a work environment. Staff play an important role in teaching and reinforcing the expectations of employers and agencies. Setting clear expectations and consequences is one of the more difficult tasks staff perform. Corps Members must adhere to a standard workplace code of conduct throughout their term of service (i.e., arriving to work on time, notifying a supervisor about an absence, having supervisors sign time sheets, etc.). Some Members have different expectations of community service; they see themselves as "volunteers" who should be able to have more flexibility in their schedules. In addition, personal difficulties such as changes in child-care provision, lack of money to pay for carfare, extreme travel distances, and family problems interfere with Corps Members' ability to follow-through with their site supervisors' expectations. Staff spend a great amount of time addressing these workplace issues, problem solving with Corps Members and, at times, resorting to levels of discipline (including suspension and termination) to provide the consistency essential to the program.

The qualities and skills of the staff needed to successfully direct and coordinate this program are unusual and varied. In any given week staff may be called upon to train Corps Members in making relevant health presentations, settle disputes between Members and their site supervisors, intervene on behalf of a Member whose benefits with AFDC have been terminated, provide counseling to a Member experiencing family difficulties, write a grant, or develop an evaluation tool for measuring impact of an asthma program for school-age children.

COMMUNITY SERVICE AS A LIFE-TRANSFORMING EXPERIENCE

It has become evident over the past four and a half years that many Members are transformed by their AmeriCorps experience. The combination of providing relevant and important community health services, being part of a supportive, respectful environment, having exposure to new ideas and topics of interest, and working in partnership with a group of people sharing an ethic of service is a profound experience. For most Corps Members, the experience helps to illuminate career goals, and their personal testimony illustrates the impact of their participation:

> With respect to my future in medicine, it provided me with exposure to primary health care on the front line. It helped me to gain more insight into what primary care is and what it should be. The Chicago Health Corps has allowed me to strengthen my interest in healthcare. I will be attending graduate school in Public Health in the fall prior to applying for medical school. I cannot stress enough how valuable my AmeriCorps experience has been.

One Corps Member ended up moving into the community he was working in.

> After a lot of the work that we did, I felt my role in my next stage as a researcher would be a lot more integrated if I actually moved into the community, started living there and start understanding what was going on. So that was part of it, becoming a community member on that side of things so that rather than the traditional model of researchers coming in, take their data, and then go back to the lab and analyze what's going on, I think I can do it from a different standpoint where I'm there, living right next to the school, so I can see what's going on. I'm a lot more in tune with it.

The experience also transforms what the term "healthcare" means to Corps Members. From this same Corps Member:

> I would say the biggest change in myself that I have seen was coming in with the concept of healthcare, and now I see you can get all the information you want, you can do all the educating you want, but if you don't understand the source, what creates the situation, your

effect and influence is really limited. To educate anybody about how to reduce hazards [of lead poisoning], or how to take precautions or do whatever, the fact is that a house that's falling apart that's been covered in lead paint all has to do with a source. Healthcare by itself, providing information isn't necessarily enough if you don't understand the context. Number one, "Why is this house covered with lead paint?" Well, let's look at the issue of lead paint, why that was still legal until a certain year. Let's look at the condition of housing. Why is somebody living in a house that's falling apart? Why is somebody living in this community? So there's really a context that I'm starting to understand a lot more of why health problems are occurring in the first place. As opposed to merely coming in with information. "OK, this is going to temporarily solve a problem." A focus on the cause, not just the solution and understanding how involved a real solution is.

Another Corps Member feels that her knowledge of PHC and community organizing has provided her with the tools to be an effective community leader.

When I first came to the Health Corps, I remember that the only thing I wanted to do was to work with teenage moms, because I was a teenage mom, and I wanted to prevent teenage pregnancy. And then as the year progressed, I decided that wasn't my main function anymore. I wanted to go out and provide health education for kids and parents, and whoever, just to let them know what "health" was, because really in underserved areas we don't know how important it is to see the doctor. We just see "doctors," we don't talk about, like, stress as being part of health. We just look at going to the doctor, getting a regular doctor check-up. And me getting the chance to provide this information to young people and parents, I think I've changed a whole lot, and I've changed my whole career goal, because I wanted to be a teacher at first, but now I'm getting ready to take my prerequisites for nursing school.

So, I've changed a whole lot. Sue [her first supervisor] says she saw me as this frantic person who just wanted to talk to teenage moms and prevent teenage pregnancies, and now she sees me as a totally different person who's out promoting health and trying to provide health education to underserved populations.

Prior to this Member's enlistment with the Health Corps, she had no community involvement but now serves on three neighborhood boards, has continued her involvement with the Youth Consortium (a project she helped organize during her term of service) and has joined her mother to organize social and religious events for children in her former neighborhood. This Member has recruited three friends into the Health Corps and is now employed by the Health Corps as a Team Leader for the Youth Health Education Team, providing supervision for eight Corps Members, and has been hired as a family interviewer for a parent-toddler study, a five-year federally funded research project.

OUTCOMES

At this writing, the Chicago Health Corps has provided 122 volunteers with the opportunity to participate in the program for a total of 103,487 hours of community service at 31 sites around the city in exchange for a minimal living allowance that roughly equals $5.15 per hour (plus health insurance, child care, and the educational benefit). Community health workers in the city of Chicago have recently unionized, and under the auspices of Local 73 of the General Service Employee Union have a negotiated rate of $9.27 per hour (after six months on the job, plus pension, welfare, and health benefits). Comparing the hourly rates, it would have cost $426,366 more for organized community workers to provide the same services that Chicago Health Corps Members have provided. In terms of real dollar amounts, the benefits negotiated for the union workers far exceed that of the Corps Members. Thus, if we were able to factor this benefit compensation into the equation, the cost savings for the services provided by the Corps Members would be seen as even more impressive.

Service hours performed by Chicago Health Corps Members have resulted in over 4,681 children being screened for lead poisoning, receiving home visits, and/or receiving health education about the toxin; the creation of community environmental awareness clubs and grassroots efforts for safer housing; services to increase capacity for self-care having been provided to 34,746 in schools, after-school clubs, and community health centers; and a total of 25,779 enabling services for women of childbearing age and their children. Most services took the form of health education about such topics as conflict resolution, HIV/AIDS awareness and prevention, personal hygiene, first aid, teen self-care, self-esteem, and breastfeeding promotion.

THE FUTURE OF THE CHICAGO HEALTH CORPS

Currently, funding of AmeriCorps programs appears to be more stable following negotiations between Congress and the Corporation for National Service; however, as with many federal programs, monies will be decreased over the next few years which will require an increase in local matching funds. The Chicago Health Corps will need to find long-term solutions to achieving sustainability. These will include increased local investment from community partners and perhaps support from the state and university. Clearly, the values and impact of this program need to be documented. Creative solutions for financing the local match can be realized. In essence, this program's future rests with the public will. If we have proved our worth to the community (and we believe we have) then local matching support will become a reality.

REFERENCES

Freire, P. *Education for critical consciousness.* New York: Seabury Press, 1973; Continuum Press, 1983 and Wallerstein, N. and Bernstein, E., Empowerment education: Freire's ideas adapted to health education. *Health Education Quarterly,* 15(4): 370–394, Winter 1988.

Hissong, T. (Producer & Director) 1997. *Primary health care: Doing something about it* (video). Available from the Centre for the Study of Primary Health Care, 845 S. Damen Ave., Chicago, IL 60612.

Hissong, T. (Producer & Director) 1997. *The Chicago Health Corps: It works* (video). Available from the Illinois Area Health Education Centers Program, 905 S. Wolcott Ave., Chicago, IL 60612.

Hope, A. & Timmel, S. (1984). *Training for transformation—a handbook for community workers.* Zimbabwe: Mambo Press.

Kretzman, J. & McKnight, J. (1993). *Building communities from the inside out.* Centers for Urban Affairs & Policy Research, Northwestern University.

McElmurry, B. J., Wansley, R., Gugenheim, A. M., Gombe, S., & Dublin, P. The Chicago Health Corps: Strengthening communities through structured volunteer service. *Advanced Practice Nursing Quarterly,* 1997, 2(4), 59–66, Aspen Publishers, Inc.

Voices for Illinois Children. (1994). *Chicago kids count: Community by community profiles of child well-being.* Chicago: Author.

Chapter 10

The Austin Community Wellness Initiative: Rebuilding Community Through Matching Capacities

JACQUELINE REED
with the assistance of
CYNTHIA TYSKA

Acknowledgments
Special acknowledgments are given to the citizen leaders who helped organize the capacity-building work and to the Kellogg Foundation for providing the funds for the Wellness Initiative. We are also extremely grateful for the ongoing support of John McKnight who has been a trusted colleague and adviser on this project.

153

How can we start seeing the positive aspects of our community and stop describing and thinking about it in negative terms—gangs, violence, drugs, corruption, public assistance, homicide rates, infant mortality rates? What are the community strengths and how can we use them as resources to rebuild the community? How can we address the reality of the negatives through the work of the positives?

In our community, people have been conditioned to believe that they do not have the power to change things, that they are clients with needs and deficiencies who should wait for some change to happen, and that professionals have the answers and resources to create the change. People stop believing in themselves—neighbors stop reaching out to neighbors—and begin to rely on professionals. This disempowers an individual's natural sense of community with others. How can individual community residents rediscover their natural powers to make a difference in themselves and in their communities?

WESTSIDE HEALTH AUTHORITY

A group of local Austin community organizations, who came together under the auspices of the Westside Health Authority, reframed their dissatisfaction with merely reacting to community problems into a commitment to become creators of change in the neighborhood. Thus, building and supporting capacities of community organizations and grassroots community people became the mission of the WHA.

Formed in 1988, the WHA sought to organize people around a common vision for the community and develop strategic plans to accomplish that vision, using the assets of community residents. It operated from the premise that it will eventually go out of business—once the vision became reality—for it is merely a "table" from which relationships between neighbors are nurtured. Once the relationships have been established, people can meet at their own kitchen table to build new dreams, and WHA's table can be folded up and put away. In the same vein, it seeks external funding and external collaborations, including university-based efforts, that fit its ideas and mission, not vice versa.

Overall, the WHA's general membership consists of a coalition of forty-one groups and individuals with varying talents and interests, largely from the Austin and West Garfield Park communities on the west side of Chicago. Membership is open to all who wish to participate from this community of 138,000 people. The members meet together at least once a month to plan and report progress on healthcare, job and economic development opportunities, research and public policy issues, and community wellness. The eleven-member board of directors, which has authority over WHA programs and staff, is elected from the general membership body. The work in each of the identified areas is carried out by an advisory group made up of citizens and professionals. For example, the health careers and wellness projects each have separate advisory boards made up of people with experience or expertise in the respective project areas. The advisory group serves to provide fresh ideas and mediate potential conflicts between WHA's staff and the board of directors (who may also be subcontractors on projects). For example, four board members are executive directors of community organizations, which have contracts with the Wellness Initiative. The Advisory Group for the Wellness Initiative consists of two community residents, a family nurse practitioner from a local health clinic, a pastor of a local Lutheran church, and a case manager.

AN AFRICAN-AMERICAN COMMUNITY ETHOS

Being helpful, useful, and giving to others was the key to resurrecting the community spirit in Austin. Reflecting upon the regular activities of people in our community, we know that there are people who take care of their families and give and give and give. Their capacity to give themselves away already existed but how could this become a community ethos? How could we help people see themselves as gifts to others in the community? How could we help them help their neighbors? The interdependence of social bonds and relationships among members of African-American churches influenced adoption of the church as a model for this community ethos. Although often situated in a dysfunctional environment, the church functions as a well community. It is able to use the resources within the church to sustain itself, and goes outside of the church only when they are unavailable from within. For example, when the church needs money, women will sell peanuts in the hot sun to raise it; when the church's physical structure needs work, there's a roofer, plumber, or electrician ready to do it. There was something going on within the Austin churches that was not going on within the broader Austin community itself. One of these things was that people in the church knew the pastor and trusted the pastor not to exploit them. But we knew that people in the Austin community did not necessarily know their neighbors and felt they could easily be exploited by one another. For example, someone's house might need painting but a neighbor will not help because the homeowner's son is a drug addict and is not doing his part. So we wanted to look at ways to address mistrust and fear of exploitation and work at ways to build bonds between neighbors, and reestablish trust and problem solving in the process.

Because the "Nguza Saba" Principles (Principles of Blackness) embody the ideas we wanted to nurture in the community, they also became part of the community ethos and guided our work in the community. These principles are: Umoja (Unity), Kujichakaglia (Self-Determination), Ujema (Collective Work and Responsibility), Ujimaa (Cooperative Economics and Familyhood), Nia (Purpose), Kuumba (Creativity), and Imani (Faith).

THE COMMUNITY WELLNESS INITIATIVE

The Wellness Initiative grew out of these motives, concerns, goals, and principles. Funded by the W. K. Kellogg Foundation during 1992–95, the Wellness

Initiative focused its resources on promoting sharing, caring, and giving among neighbors as a means of rebuilding the health and well-being of the Austin/West Garfield Park communities and its 138,000 residents. This paper discusses one major component of the initiative.

CAPACITY BUILDING THROUGH ASSET ORGANIZING

Utilizing McKnight and Kretzmann's (1990) community capacity building model, two of the Wellness Initiative's objectives were to: (1) identify an inventory of "gifts" of Austin and West Garfield Park community residents; and (2) develop a system of "gifts" to be shared.

Kretzmann and McKnight (1993) discussed their asset-based community development process as one which built upon what already exists in the community, and which depends upon agenda building, problem solving and relationship-building capacities, and strengths of local residents, local associations, and local institutions, identifying the latter three as the major categories of community-based assets. "The key to neighborhood regeneration, then, is to locate all of the available local assets, to begin connecting them with one another in ways that multiply their power and effectiveness, and to begin harnessing those local institutions that are not yet available for local development purposes" (Kretzmann & McKnight, 1993, p. 4). In the Wellness Initiative, WHA focused its energies on assets of individuals in the community, and collaborated with John McKnight of Northwestern University in developing an asset organizing component.

Connectors. Several community residents were hired and trained to visit with other community residents to identify the skills and capacities they possessed. The Capacity Inventory developed by McKnight and Kretzmann (1990) was the tool initially used to aid in this process. The inventory consists of a list of 174 items in addition to nineteen short-response, open-ended questions. Categories cover skills, hobbies, group affiliations, and job experience. Examples of some of the listed items, to which individuals indicated they did or did not have skill or experience, are: fixing leaky faucets, painting, mowing lawns, electrical repairs, repairing automobiles, planting and caring for gardens, caring for children, taking children on field trips, preparing meals for large numbers of people, making a budget, taking phone messages, keeping track of supplies, and driving a car.

Although we acquired over eight hundred completed inventories, the inventory document was abandoned and replaced with story collection after a year, primarily because the inventory interfered with forming relationships between the connector and the potential gift giver. We also realized that even though the inventory provided information about one's capacity it did not provide information on one's character, which we believe is necessary to connect gift givers and recipients. In addition, the acquisition of data proved to be insufficient for matching people, so the project's focus shifted from collecting information on assets to collecting information on matches. Story collection involved residents in discussions about their lives, what they did, what they liked to do, and what their home and job skills were. It elicited information that was needed for the inventory plus valuable information about who these community residents really were and how we could best match them with each other. Gift-givers' stories were recorded on forms McKnight's staff developed for that purpose. This shift in the gift-seeking process resulted in three kinds of matching during the three-year period: individual-to-individual, individual-to-group, and group/association formation.

Individual-to-Individual Matches

Matching the right people together and sustaining those relationships as a means of building trust and spreading the word was more important than getting large quantities of matches. But several dozen individual-to-individual matches were made, with some neighbors providing extremely valuable services to others who were recruited from groups formed by the connectors, block organizing, and other group means. Some neighbors shared transportation, some shared clothing, and some shared demanding responsibilities:

- A woman took in a neighbor and her three children for several months
- An unemployed, skilled man was taken in by a neighbor who provided food and shelter in exchange for plastering and electrical work
- Children from alcoholic parents were matched with surrogate parents in the community
- A neighbor helped a paraplegic with shopping
- A gang member's match with a postal worker helped him get a job. Several maladaptive and abusive family members of this gang affiliate have become active in job searching and positive activities as a result of this match.
- A newly released, homeless ex-offender was matched with an adjusted ex-offender for support and counseling, and as a result was provided shelter and support until he could establish himself.
- A gunshot victim was matched with a mother grieving for her son who had been shot

The matches have made tremendous impact on lives. For example, gang members and drug dealers gained greater respect and appreciation for community residents. When they saw several members actively involved with the Wellness Initiative reaching out to them, it changed their attitude toward drug dealing. It seemed to us that as they became aware of how their behavior affected others, they knew the residents by name, and in the end cared what those neighbors thought of them. In addition, those who have been helped are reaching out to their peers. The gunshot victim is mentoring another gunshot victim; several gang members who were abusive to their girlfriends are pressuring other gang members to desist from abusing their female companions. The ripple effect of these interactions is seen in the neighborhood, but not easily counted.

Individual-to-Group Matches

This component consisted of connecting people who wanted to contribute their gift in a structured environment where they would not be overwhelmed and be assured of more control. To use their capacity, a connector would refer them to community organizations that provided services related to the gift-giver's skills. The initial component of the Adopt-a-Grandparent group (discussed later) started out with a connection with a local hospital that identified such a need. Sewing groups formed in the same way where gift givers could either teach or learn sewing.

These matches had mixed results. While this was a major focus initially as the wellness connectors sought to place gift givers, many of the organizations had too many encumbrances to use the gifts. For example, agencies required training and/or certification for volunteers and often did not have sufficient flexibility within their structure to use volunteers.

Group Connections and Associations Formed

Organizing people in groups was a major strategy used to address the fear of being exploited and to enhance group identity and support. The group was also seen as a means of sustaining the work after the staff support left.

Two self-help groups were formed during the project. **Parents Anonymous** was organized by a young woman with six children who was distraught with hearing all the horror stories about child abuse/neglect that exists even in foster homes. Six parents meet weekly and although the group has not grown, they find tremendous support from each other. A volunteer child-care worker supervises their children during their meetings. **Women's Alcoholics Anonymous Group** was organized at WHA by women who wanted a program specifically related to their needs. The group meets weekly with strong participation and leadership.

Wellness Workers. One of the more successful groups—Wellness Workers—provides gifts to children, teens, the elderly, and the community at large. Comprised of unemployed, many highly skilled, men who participate in the Earnfare Program, it is a state-run program which assists individuals in getting off of general assistance. Many of these participants are alienated from the community because of drug usage or other problems, but saw their involvement with the Wellness Initiative as a means of re-entering the community and regaining community respect. Among the activities their volunteerism supports are the following:

- Monitoring school halls at local high schools to reduce delinquent behavior
- Tutoring young children in math and English
- Supervising the playlot (former hot spot for drug dealers) adjacent to WHA's building
- Assisting the Boy Scouts and 4-H leaders
- Doing errands/chores for seniors and single parents

All events celebrating community gift giving were organized and facilitated by these Wellness Workers. Their families came to these events and new self-images were created that helped many workers regain their respect. As a result, all of the participants made greater efforts at reducing their consumption of illicit drugs and alcohol and several found employment. Feedback from family members has been inspiring. For example, one wife was astounded to find her husband not only coming home on payday—which he seldom did before—but also carrying a bag of food purchased on his first solo trip to the grocery store.

Children Connections. Some of the most successful areas were connecting adults with children and connecting teens and elderly citizens or older teens and younger teens. Residents see children as vulnerable and trustworthy of gifts even when their parents may not be. Three of these major connections are as follows:

- A 4-H Club was formed with several parents supporting over 67 children, meeting weekly, often twice weekly (the only 4-H club on Chicago's west side)
- A Boy Scout troop was formed—for the first time in twelve years— and maintained by four community volunteers
- A community group of parents calling themselves Parents' Advisory Council (PAC) supports and facilitates the Kiddie Core Community (KCC), a group of over forty children, many of whom are neglected by their parents.

Activities in the 4-H Club and Boy Scouts have been consistent with the traditional actvities of these clubs. KCC activities were planned and resourced entirely by the PAC and include after-school tutoring, Black history projects, personal hygiene and grooming, leadership development, and gift-sharing opportunities for the youth.

Teen Connections. Three unique characteristics present an opportunity for elderly residents to connect with teens: The elderly have more available time, are willing to take more risk since they are unable or unwilling to leave the neighborhood, and have a need to tell their stories as part of their psychosocial development. Seven groups evolved from the connections made between teenagers and senior citizens in the community. Two of these programs are described here:

- *Adopt-a-Grandparent.* Twelve African-American high school students connected with mostly white, convalescing seniors at a bordering suburban, WHA-member hospital that was seeking ways to reach out and integrate more with the Austin community. By integrating an identified hospital staff person in this effort, the program became sustainable.
- *Intergenerational Group.* Nine seniors were matched with twenty-two students for support and enhancement. The seniors shared their stories of struggle and about their youth and times in which they grew up; for example, when they first picked cotton, and what it felt like to see "For Colored" signs. And the students taught the seniors what it feels like when

teachers really do not care, which was a revelation for seniors today. Additional grant funds provided support for students' senior interviews to be printed and disseminated as stories. Over four hundred manuscripts have been distributed. One local high school teacher used the manuscript in his history class. The seniors also went to the schools to teach history classes.

LESSONS LEARNED

Most of our lessons learned reflect the unpredictability of working in communities. The methodology we used to approach asset-based organizing was heavily influenced by our observations of the church as a model and the work of John McKnight. Asset-based organizing is new and challenges many traditional ways of community development, but we did not anticipate the degree to which these traditions were ingrained into everyday community life and organizational behavior.

Based on standard methods for implementing a project, WHA developed various tools to not only evaluate the project but also to assist in the work process. A significant amount of time was spent on developing the right kind of survey, only later to be discarded. We also developed a data base for connecting people with certain kinds of assets with those in need—this too was inadequate. Connecting people to assist each other in the community proved to be more challenging than merely having the right concept or the right tool. The challenge was to build relationships between the organization and people and to build trust among neighbors. Most of our lessons learned center around defining, clarifying, and enhancing these personal relationships among people. Here are some of our learnings.

1. The effort to make contact with people and identify and use their capacities was not easily understood, and because of this was sometimes hindered by the connector's own tendency to render the care. Soliciting residents' cooperation as partners in rebuilding their communities had to be constantly redefined in interactions with them, not only because of their fear and mistrust of others but also because of their dependency on professional services. When residents were approached, their first reactions were to focus on needs and deficiencies and ways to address them that only a professional could implement; they did not see themselves as the source of the "solutions." For example, residents talked about the need for more police to address the gang issue and/or more parenting programs to help neglectful parents. While they envisioned a role for themselves as advocates for such changes by mobilizing and pressuring the city to address gang violence or referring parents to the child abuse hotline, they could not see a role for themselves in directly intervening in gang-related activities or nurturing others families.

2. Well-established organizations known for specific services or organizing to "fight an enemy" can be a hindrance to asset-based organizing. It is difficult to change the old patterns of working in the community especially

when new approaches are unfamiliar and bear uncertain outcomes. It is easier for an organization to revert back to familiar and more comfortable behaviors which demonstrate something has been "done" rather than work on the new behavior of "building relationships" whose outcomes are not always as tangible as the old ones. In addition, community residents perceive the organizations through their well-established identities and not as facilitators of something new and, accordingly, inadvertently reinforce the organization's old patterns.

3. It is difficult to organize people to use their assets without being able to specifically discuss the needs for their assets if the need is not yet apparent. For example, when a connector found enthusiastic support from a neighbor through door knocking, it was difficult to know what to do with the offer because you do not always have a person who needs the kind of help that is being offered. Waiting to accept an offer of help gives the illusion that you do not really need the neighbor's assistance. It became more productive for the project to bring neighborhood people together on their own blocks and let group interactions take place naturally. Through this approach, people often built their own relationships and subsequently offered assistance to each other, thus rebuilding a helping community ethos on their own.

4. Identifying, nurturing, and supporting the talents of potential leaders is important to capacity building in neighborhoods. We need to build structures to support the diversity of talent these leaders have. Many talented people who wanted to assist in community building did not feel capable and/or were not interested in planning. On the other hand, some leaders who had an interest in planning may also have had hidden agendas (e.g., gaining political support for an office). Additional resources need to be devoted to address these concerns.

5. Identifying and sustaining community leadership is difficult and continues to be a major obstacle for the organization. Leaders often look to organizations for direction and support and without adequate staff they burn out or give up. In addition, while heavy demands are placed on leaders, there is little reward from the community for their untiring efforts.

6. Volunteers who are not gainfully employed elsewhere sought job-related benefits with the Wellness Initiative. Some participants joined groups because they could derive benefits such as self-esteem, support for a new lifestyle, job leads and directions, and mentoring from peers. However, often the group process itself falsely raised their job expectations. Many thought they would find jobs if they started to do the "right thing."

SUSTAINABILITY

Several of the groups that targeted youth are continuing to meet without staff involvement. The 4-H club won a state championship, and the Boy Scout troop and the Kiddie Core Community have also stabilized. The most promising group is one composed of residents from twenty blocks in the community who recently mobilized themselves around the concept of "it takes a village to raise a child." While it is too early to assess how effective the capacity building scheme will work in this group, the effort demonstrates how citizen leaders are taking hold of their vision and using their own resources to rebuild their neighborhoods. This work holds much promise for continuing WHAs Wellness Initiative.

Economic Benefits. As a result of organizing assets, certain economic development benefits were realized. Wellness Workers who had participated in home repairs organized themselves into a handyman business. Until the business could be "hatched" and become self-supporting, WHA provided initial support with free office space, photocopying, and telephone service. Now self-supporting, the business is regularly employed by local residents and churches.

Students from two local high schools connected to local hospitals by selling crafts in their gift shops. The students now operate their own businesses in craft stores they opened at their own schools. As another example, in the play-lot next door to WHA, children under the age of ten operate a snow cone stand during the summer months, transforming the aura of the lot from the negative economy of drug dealing that once occurred there to the hopeful economy of a young entrepreneur's dreams.

Benefits of Collaboration. One benefit is related to the community organizations themselves. Formerly organized around issues, WHA community organizations have largely abandoned them and now almost exclusively focus on capacity building. The success of their wellness projects surprised many executives and the structure and learning provided by this initiative opened new pathways for community organizing. However, since both issue organizing and capacity building are needed in community development, the challenge has now become how to balance the two in such efforts. The second benefit of collaboration focuses on the project funder and university collaborator. Both were open and flexible enough to allow major changes in the project which in turn resulted in a project that fit the community. These are all necessary conditions for sustainability.

THE WELL COMMUNITY

The idea of the Wellness Initiative was to build a campaign that promoted self and mutual help which could be sustained. Relationship quantity was secondary to relationship quality and to how the relationships added to the overall fabric of the community in the long run. It is very reassuring to us that even after the funding has ended people are still organized and helping each other. It is through this effort that responsible citizenship is being redefined and communities rebuilt. The building of relationships is the critical first step in forming communities. Vision and systemic change are realized through relationships. People have to be at the forefront of a democratic system; their involvement cannot be replaced by outside experts using data and/or special interests which influence so much of public policy today. Most people in the community have real concerns about the child welfare, public welfare, health-care, and criminal justice systems, but have little confidence in their current practices. Building a community vision that uses assets that are interconnected with these systems will not only lead to sustainable community changes but will also reaffirm the credibility of democracy for people who have too long been disengaged from the process.

REFERENCES

Kretzmann, J. P. & McKnight, J. L. (1993). *Building communities from the inside out: A path toward finding and mobilizing a community's assets.* Chicago: ACTA Publications.

McKnight, J. L. & Kretzmann, J. (1990). *Mapping community capacity.* Evanston, IL: Institute for Policy Research.

Chapter 11

Primary Health Care in an Urban Teaching Community Health Center

ELLEN BARTON
with the assistance of
CYNTHIA TYSKA

Acknowledgments
Sincerest thanks to the following who taught about the strengths of the community, the importance of public health outside of clinic walls, and the resiliency of the human spirit: Jackie Reed, MS; Sarah Groves, RN; Dr.PH.; Naomi Ervin; RN, Ph.D.; Len Sharber, M.Div.; Terry O'Neal, RN, MA; and Judy Cooksey, MD, MPH.

INTRODUCTION

How one develops one's role in an organization and how that organization develops its culture and orientation toward the people it serves are primary indicators of how successfully those people are served. Community health centers in underserved urban areas are challenged with presenting, delivering, or providing healthcare to constituents who live in sometimes unstable, turbulent community contexts. Such contexts can be so overwhelming for individuals, families, and groups that any kind of healthcare is perceived as inadequate in the provider's mind. What ingredients are needed to be effective in the role of healthcare provider under these circumstances?

There are probably an infinite number of ingredients that will prove successful in working with underserved communities. The combination shared here is what I, as a healthcare professional, developed for myself as a result of my personal philosophy, professional training and experiences, and my work within a continuously responsive community health center. As a certified family nurse practitioner with advanced practice in public health issues, I was fully prepared for direct service with patients, addressing broader issues of epidemiology and prevention, and addressing patients' community environments through community assessments and program planning and evaluation. The perspective of primary health care (PHC) along with the notion of capacity building came to complete my philosophy of what healthcare is and how I wanted to deliver it. As a healthcare provider, education director, and leader focusing on an individual's health as well as the context of that health, I sought to achieve, directly or indirectly:

- Effective community contexts and development
- Reality-based health professions education and research
- Comprehensive and accessible health services for all populations
- Services that address health promotion and disease prevention
- Patient partnerships that address health, social, and economic issues
- Community-based foci and efforts that include views toward policy development

COMMUNITY CONTEXT AND DEVELOPMENT

Through the filter of community development, health is viewed as an outgrowth of social, political, and economic conditions that individuals, families, groups, and communities experience (Soares, Swider, & McElmurry, 1999). Health planning and improvement efforts are therefore a result of individuals, families, groups, and communities acting alone and in concert to affect structural changes in their environments. I concur with Soares, Swider, and McElmurry (1999) that these changes can occur because community residents already possess (or can acquire) the skills necessary to improve the health of their community. Further, it is important that this philosophy be shared by both the nurse practitioner and the stated goals of the community health center in which he/she works.

Effective PHC requires that care in a clinical setting is delivered beyond individuals to extended families, groups, and communities. Healthcare delivery in medically underserved areas requires unique strategies for handling patients' complex social and medical problems, harnessing strengths within families, and creating effective networks among various programs and communities. It also requires effective communication, individualized patient teaching, preventive services, and connecting patients with public health services within their own communities.

As a medically underserved Chicago community, Austin provides a complex and challenging context for a community health center trying to make a difference. Located on Chicago's west side, Austin is primarily an African-American community consisting of many young families, many children, and a high birth rate. A large percentage of the population is on public assistance, but there is also a large middle class. Austin is a medically underserved area with a preponderance of serious health problems such as lead poisoning, sexually transmitted diseases, tuberculosis, early death due to asthma, cardiovascular disease, homicides, and accidents. The strengths of the community reside with extended families, neighborhood connections, block clubs, community organizations, social service agencies, and its large number of churches.

THE COMMUNITY HEALTH CENTER

Circle Family Care (CFC) is a Federally Qualified Health Center (FQHC) which has provided holistic healthcare within Austin and two other Chicago communities (Humboldt Park and West Garfield) since 1978. This community-based organization was formed to provide holistic primary care to the urban poor by providing medical care, counseling, and spiritual care to patients. Through this holistic model, CFC personnel partner with patients, their families, and community organizations to improve health and uplift the community spirit. CFC is committed to the Austin community, and many of its healthcare providers and administrators are not only familiar with neighborhood issues but are also Austin residents. Collaborative, interdisciplinary relationships exist among CFC's physicians, nurse practitioners, clinical pharmacists, nurses, pastoral counselors, and case managers who all work together to improve patient care. The center's services include women's health, adult health, well child care and prenatal care, an HIV Early Intervention Project, and a mobile health team which provides primary care in shelters (e.g., general physicals, TB screening, chronic illness treatment, well child care). A lead abatement program helps families find housing during lead removal from their homes, provides public education on treatment, prevention of lead poisoning, and also assists in advocacy. CFC's counseling division also provides foster care services, parenting classes, and individual/family counseling.

REALITY-BASED EDUCATION AND RESEARCH

In 1994, CFC formed an educational affiliation with the University of Illinois at Chicago (UIC). One of the goals of this Teaching Community Health

Center (TCHC) affiliation is to help change the health professions' training focus from hospital settings to urban community health centers in medically underserved communities. When students spend the majority of their learning time in settings where the principles of community-oriented primary care, cross cultural focus, strong communication skills, and empathy are emphasized, they become better prepared and motivated to work in medically underserved areas. This kind of training ultimately increases the number of skilled and committed healthcare providers needed to work in community-based healthcare in medically underserved communities. For the Austin community this means that there is an increase in both the amount of available, quality primary care and access to it.

Educational experiences in an urban clinic should have instructional merit but should also serve a useful purpose for the agency so that both student and clinic derive benefits from the experience and neither can be construed as a drain upon the other. For health professions students, CFC's education director emphasizes *doing* case management, not just thinking and learning about it. Accordingly, health professions students have worked on projects in the clinic which improve CFC clinical care such as prenatal and asthma education, organizing a resource directory, managed care education, and community assessment. These are practical rather than theoretical pieces that can be used by the clinic staff after a student's departure.

A second goal of the CFC/UIC affiliation is the use of a multidisciplinary approach in promoting comprehensive PHC. This fits with CFC personnel's philosophy of moving away from problem-oriented care to keeping people healthy and functioning well within their communities.

The third goal of the TCHC affiliation is the development of a community-based model where community agencies, residents, and CFC clients are all part of the center's decision-making process that addresses community health issues and methods for problem solving. Services extend beyond individual clients to interactions with community organizations and activities. An organizational partnership is created between the community and our institutions to encourage planned and consistent institutional responsiveness to community needs.

Reality-Based Research

The educational center contains resource directories, demographics, health statistics, and Internet linkages which all community partners can share. Part of UIC's educational affiliation is to bring technical assistance and information to the community. In my capacity as the education director, I act as a liaison and disseminate the information that comes into the center. For example, my objectives are to assist CFC management, influence policy makers where I can, increase UIC faculty and student interest in implementing service-oriented projects (such as demonstrations or evaluations), and summarize relevant information. Research requests are always framed within the context of giving CFC something it needs: doing research that helps the community, improving care at CFC, or contributing to program evaluation. The center also asks for respect of staff members' time: We do not want research clogging up the clinic with extra work or requirements that impede the normal flow of healthcare practice at the clinic. Research is limited to what agency personnel deem appropriate or useful to the center. CFC also has a research committee that sets and follows certain guidelines for acceptable research which include utility, appropriateness, confidentiality, unobtrusiveness, and time efficiency.

Useful Research

What is the point of doing research if it is off the mark? University researchers meet with community providers to develop research in areas of concern identified by the community. Generally, relevant areas of research include public health, preventive healthcare, patient compliance, quality assurance, and cost-effectiveness. Future research projects may involve partnering with universities for assistance in proposal writing, evaluating programs, assisting community agencies' funding searches, developing curriculum for the TCHC, and creating literature reviews to increase the knowledge flow from the university to the center.

COMPREHENSIVE AND ACCESSIBLE CARE

The personnel in a comprehensive healthcare center like CFC know and effectively use community resources. Available community resources are potential partners who can combine knowledge and resources to strengthen community services. CFC staff also developed and use a resource manual for the Austin community to better facilitate patient referrals. The manual covers the following areas: education, churches, community organizations, counseling, day care, public information, health services, legal services, managed care, nutrition, pregnancy, family planning, senior citizen services, substance abuse treatment, economic, housing, and training issues.

Accessible healthcare reflects a holistic approach that goes beyond the boundaries of the clinic to incorporate a larger concept of community in the delivery of service, problem-solving and capacity building. In developing effective PHC, it helps to provide outreach activities where people congregate (such as health fairs). This approach not only helps to educate healthcare providers about what is really happening in communities, but also helps to break down the mystique that surrounds medicine among community residents. By decentralizing where healthcare is provided—schools, parks, shelters, churches—access to PHC is enhanced. This approach draws in a population that would not ordinarily visit a health clinic for any reason.

PREVENTION

Prevention strategies are essential to delivering high-quality primary care, and one facet of this approach is to look beyond the presenting concern or problem.

For example, if on a well-child visit a parent is observed to be wheezing, that issue should be addressed as well as the child's health because a parent cannot effectively take care of her child if her own condition is compromised.

Prevention strategies used in a community health center should be based on an assessment of community needs. For example, if the housing structures in the community are relatively new, lead paint and pipes will not be present. Thus, lead screening would not be a priority for a community health center's prevention strategy. By examining the kind of epidemiology of a community, appropriate screening and interventions can be targeted. In Austin, lead exposure is an issue and many CFC cases involve lead poisoning in children. Through CFC staff efforts, parents become aware of housing conditions that cause lead poisoning and receive information when their children become mobile in the house. Parents learn when to get their children screened for lead poisoning and what to do if lead poisoning is found. They also learn how to advocate with their landlord or the Chicago Department of Public Health (CDPH) if abatement problems occur.

The epidemiology of the community helps the healthcare provider know which risk factors are important for screening. For example, we screen for violence as a risk factor during high school physicals. Factors such as gang affiliation, drug use, plans for the future, and conflict resolution are topics which are appropriately discussed within a prevention-oriented physical. Parents are included in this discussion and feel both supported by the healthcare provider and relieved that topics such as these are included as a part of "health." Violence factors are generally screened in the health history assessment with such questions as, "Do you feel safe in your neighborhood?" and, "Do you have a handgun in the home?" Discussing the attendant safety issues of having a handgun in the home and making referrals to community policing groups are interventions which can be done within a primary care visit.

PATIENT PARTNERSHIPS

A caring, welcoming attitude regards patients as partners in the decision-making process concerning their health. Establishing long-term relationships with healthcare providers is necessary for assisting families in maintaining or improving their health so that patients know what to watch for in their particular situations and know who they can rely on for healthcare assistance. Through this relationship, patients become knowledgeable about what they need to do to enhance their health status.

We try to form relationships that are acceptable to patients and their families and to provide interventions that are realistic and sensitive to the realities of their lives. Providing specific information, a comfortable discussion environment, considerations for a patient's life context, and focusing on patient needs and priorities gives both care giver and patient a strong foundation for building an effective partnership. For example, sexual risk reduction behavior is more than being informed about condom use; it also includes exploring issues of assertiveness, alternative behaviors to sexuality, and emotions within relationships between sexual partners. Removing sutures from an assault-related laceration also involves providing information on organizations working on violence prevention (i.e., community policing, community organizing groups, block clubs, etc.) making domestic violence referrals, and/or discussing strategies for problem solving or conflict resolution.

ADDRESSING SOCIAL AND ECONOMIC ISSUES

Effective PHC means looking beyond the individual's physical health concerns to their emotional and spiritual needs as well as life aspirations and goals. Discussing a person's life aspirations and goals with them leads to rich discussions about their interests, plans, and life's difficulties. Such activities help to boost an individual's self-confidence and help that person look toward a more economically secure future. Focusing on social and economic issues broadens the health impact toward factors which truly affect the basic health of families. Approaches CFC personnel have used include:

- Encouraging individuals to graduate from high school, discussing different career paths and how to find out about them, and letting them know about available financial aid.
- Having relevant information readily available for patients who are engaged in job placement efforts and training programs.
- Discussing personal strengths such as problem solving, assertiveness, budgeting, communication, and organization.

COMMUNITY-BASED EFFORTS

To provide effective PHC, programs and activities need to be based on community priorities as well as epidemiology and statistics. Generalized information derived from clinical experiences can be channeled to advisory boards to better inform leaders and plan community initiatives.

Some of the highest rates of sexually transmitted diseases (STDs) exist in the Austin and Garfield Park communities. To address this issue, the District Health Council sponsored two forums (epidemiology and treatment of STDs, and multifaceted strategies for successful risk reduction) which gathered community providers, case managers, social service workers, school personnel, and community leaders. These forums lead to coordinated services among community health clinics and the development of a culturally appropriate public education risk reduction program for schools and the community at large.

Another example of community responsiveness centers on barriers Medicaid patients experience from managed care marketing abuses. During the transition to MediPlan Plus (the Illinois managed care program for Medicaid recipients), patients are enrolled in HMOs with incomplete and often misleading information. Patients are told they can continue to see their current healthcare provider when, in fact, they often cannot. Further, patients are told that their level of care will be exactly the same if they change healthcare plans when that is rarely the case. Patients who have received continuous care from CFC are now being assigned to HMOs far outside their geographical living area, which presents travel and time barriers that compromise a patient's compliance with good continuity of care. Families we have followed for five years now do not know the location of their HMO provider. In this scenario, profits come before care; this is patient exploitation.

We provide patients with specific information about resigning from such programs if they are dissatisfied with them, and encourage them to file incidence reports with the Illinois Department of Public Aid (IDPA). In an effort to affect changes on a system-wide level, we also share these experiences with responsible authorities and community leaders. For example, the Campaign for Better Healthcare and the Westside Health Authority involved both healthcare providers and patients in providing testimonial feedback to the IDPA and Illinois policy makers on this issue during the hearings on MediPlan Plus.

POLICY DEVELOPMENT

At CFC, primary care providers act in an advisory role to boards such as the District Health Councils or the Westside Health Authority (Reed, 1999). Committee work with the latter has included the Wellness Initiative where community capacity building has involved connecting people to community intervention, and larger issues such as crime and economic development that enhance citizen participation and strengthen neighborhoods.

By targeting issues that affect the community, population-based strategies can be developed. Issues from the front line of healthcare that develop within a clinic and in the streets are communicated to policy makers and researchers and are eventually used to train future healthcare providers. An example of this effort is the Communicable Disease Subcommittee of the District Health Council. Austin and West Garfield have high rates of gonorrhea and chlamydia, but no public health clinic to assist in screening and treatment. Community health providers are concerned that many patients do not have access to STD screening and treatment services. A group of concerned citizens, community health providers, and CDPH administrators met to determine strategies for increasing community capacity for providing walk-in STD services to medically indigent patients. This coalition was formed within the organizing framework of the District Health Council and Westside Health Authority, and included representation from three hospital-based outpatient clinics, a community health center, a nursing center, two large public clinics, and CDPH. The outcome of this relationship-building effort and community advocacy is a CDPH STD clinic targeted for a January 1998 opening in Austin.

As CFC's education director, I advise several health policy groups, including the Committee on Environmental Justice, which was formed with a grant from the National Institute for Environmental Health for the purpose of increasing communication among researchers, providers, and community people. My role on this committee allows me to voice suggestions to improve patient care strategies for those whose health is compromised by asthma and lead presence, both problems disproportionately represented in the Austin community. The identification and alteration of environmental risk factors facilitates better patient management of their asthma or improved lead poisoning prevention. As a provider, I disseminate information to the committee to provide better care and develop connections among community agencies, advocates, and providers and thus strengthen the level and quality of healthcare. In my role as consultant, I share my experiences as a nurse practitioner in the clinic and my continuing efforts to link primary care services with broader health initiatives within the community.

Another important issue in the community is crime, especially gun violence, drug dealing, and substance abuse. Aside from the direct health effects on those involved, there are a lot of other people walking around in fear, "shell shocked," or experiencing post-traumatic stress disorder because of the homicides or near hits they have witnessed or experienced. Many families are touched by violence, having lost family members or neighbors to homicides.

Such circumstances clearly take a toll on the community's health, and these issues need to be addressed at the policy level. When gun availability decreases and gun usage penalties increase, then the fatal or crippling effects of gun-related crimes will be abated. In addition, many strategies will need to coalesce to solve the overall violence problem in communities. These strategies should include, but not be limited to, more effective policing (such as community policing) addressing violent behavior through teaching alternative problem-solving skills, providing good educational and job opportunities, and strengthening neighborhoods through economic development. When communities consistently experience such life-enhancing factors, the pull of the streets will be weakened and the epidemic of violence will dissipate.

CONCLUSION

A community health center can be an ideal environment to achieve PHC. In such a setting, PHC can be implemented in ways that allow for community, university, and policy involvement as well as good clinical practice in primary care. Additionally, the provision of wellness/prevention services, social, emotional, and spiritual support, and the clarification of personal career and education goals make such a facility invaluable to the population it serves. A community health center in a medically underserved urban area where the population experiences a wide variety of life stressors can capacity build in ways that fortify the community while fulfilling healthcare delivery goals. Led by an organizational philosophy and vision, as well as guidelines and plans for decisions and actions, dedicated individuals within an organization like CFC are able to practice within their scope of expertise and interests, yet take advantage of opportunities for external change. The organization is permeable (responsive to external influences, whether community, university, or political) yet not over-whelmed or taken over by stakeholders' interests, and still achieves a balance which serves patients, students, and community. Within the organization, inter-actions with patients and students result in "teachable moments" that may pos-itively change individual lives in ways that are difficult to capture as tangible program outcomes.

The structure of a PHC program recognizes the importance of ensuring opportunities for everyone as well as outreach to those not fully served by the healthcare community. Through CFC's Teaching Community Health Center, capacity building is fostered in the development of patients, students, and community. CFC's health services are accessible to all populations; emphasize disease prevention and health promotion; and address high-priority health concerns for community residents and the health system. Health development is integrated with overall social, educational, and economic development. CFC is a community health center that clearly illustrates PHC tenets.

REFERENCES

Soares, C., Swider, S. M., & McElmurry, B. J. (1999). *The training of commu-nity health advocates for urban United States communities: A program eval-uation.* In B. J. McElmurry, C. Tyska, & R. S. Parker (Eds.), *Primary health care in urban communities.* Boston: Jones & Bartlett.

Reed, J. (1999). *The Austin Community Wellness Initiative: Rebuilding com-munity through matching capacities.* In B. J. McElmurry, C. Tyska, & R. S. Parker (Eds.), *Primary health care in urban communities.* Boston: Jones & Bartlett.

Chapter 12

Building Healthy Latino Communities

LORI RAMOS
ROSARIO SANCHEZ
FRANCISCO RAMOS

Acknowledgments:

We acknowledge the many individuals, institutions, and foundations who have provided moral and financial support to our community health promoters, especially:

AETNA Foundation; AIDS Foundation of Chicago; Alivio Medical Center Midwifery Department; Foundation for Health Enhancement; The Chicago Community Trust; Chicago Department of Public Health—Division of HIV/AIDS Programs and Policies; Chicago Foundation for Women; Chicago Tribune Holiday Fund; Claretian Missionaries and Fr. Richard Bartlett; Crossroads Fund; The Dominican Sisters, Springfield, IL; Erie Family Health Center; GATX Corporation; Eva Hernandez, RN, MSN; The March of Dimes Birth Defects Foundation; John McNeany, CPA; National Committee on the Self-Development of People—Presbyterian Church USA; Newman's Own Fund; Opening Doors: Reducing Socio-Cultural Barriers to Health Care—A Joint Program of the Robert Wood Johnson and Kaiser Family Foundations; Presbyterian Hunger Program; The Presiding Bishop's Fund, Episocopal Church; Saint Vincent DePaul Church, Fort Wayne, IN; Sisters of St. Joseph, Philadelphia, PA; University of Illinois at Chicago College of Nursing; Beverly J. McElmurry, Ed.D, FAAN, Randy Spreen Parker, RN, Ph.D., and Janet Holden, Ph.D., University of Illinois at Chicago School of Public Health; University of Illinois at Chicago Department of Emergency Medicine; the Vineyard Christian Fellowship, Santa Monica, CA; Today's Chicago Woman Foundation; The Northern Trust; Julio Becerra; José Arrom; Corrinne Peterson; The Louis Lurie Foundation; and Greater Chicago Food Depository.

Since 1991, Centro San Bonifacio has been working to organize and mobilize health promotion projects in the West Town area of Chicago. Centro San Bonifacio was formed as a community-based organization in response to the closure of the St. Bonifacio parish in 1990 which resulted in the dispersement of over 1,400 Spanish-speaking families. Our founding board consisted of a group of Latino families who believed that the loss of their parish constituted the loss of a community center that for many years had been responsive to the needs of a large Latino population. This group of families had been meeting together as *Comunidades Eclesiales de Base* (Base Christian Communities) in their homes for over two years. Because the tradition of Base Communities in Latin America is rooted in social analysis, social justice, community self-empowerment, and mutual support, the closing of the parish inspired the members of the communities to act. Hence, the underlying theme in the founding of Centro San Bonifacio was grounded in the belief that the main protagonists in health promotion should be community members themselves.

COMMUNITY HEALTH PROMOTER TRAINING

This underlying theme motivated Centro San Bonifacio's organizers to direct all activities and projects toward self-empowerment, self-sufficiency, and leadership development in the Hispanic community. A strong commitment to peer health promotion through the training of neighborhood residents as community health promoters (CHPs) was also reflected in the programs. Centro San Bonifacio's health promoters usually begin their training with a 45-hour course in health promotion and disease prevention conducted entirely in Spanish. We offer the training twice a year and advertise it primarily through word-of-mouth and personal invitations. The average number of participants is between ten and fifteen community residents and the only requirement for graduation is attendance; thus, it is accessible as a "first step" to becoming a health promoter.

Participants in the CHP course are typically newly immigrated Latin American women, predominately from Mexico but also from Peru, Guatemala, Ecuador, and Puerto Rico. The majority of participants include homemakers, factory workers, and welfare recipients. Although most of the participants who attend the course have low literacy skills, physicians, nurses, and social workers who were trained in their native countries and immigrated to the United States have used the training program as a bridge to entering the healthcare system. The diversity of participants presents an ongoing challenge to the discussion of health-related topics in a manner that is useful and meaningful to everyone.

The CHP training curriculum is organized and implemented by a team of staff and volunteer CHPs. Initially the training workshops were provided by Spanish-speaking professionals working in their fields of expertise; however, over time CHPs have assumed more teaching responsibility. Currently, 80 percent of the curriculum is taught by CHPs.

The curriculum was originally developed and tailored to the specific health concerns of Latinos in the United States. Health statistics demonstrate that Latinos have higher rates of chronic diseases, accidents, domestic violence, and teen pregnancy (Chicago Department of Public Health, 1995; Novell, Wise, & Kleiman, 1991). Latino women are among the fastest growing risk groups for HIV/AIDS infection, and are at much higher risk for acute depression (Chicago Department of Public Health, 1995; Council on Scientific Affairs, 1991; Diaz et al., 1993). Moreover, Latinos have less access to health services, health insurance coverage, and health education (McFarlane, 1996). Based on the statisitcs, and an ongoing evaluation process which includes graduates of the course, the curriculum currently includes presentations, discussion, and popular education activities focused on the following topics:

- History of community health promoters: A global perspective
- Substance abuse and treatment
- Domestic violence
- Chronic illnesses
- Nutrition and healthy cooking
- Human sexuality
- Maternal/child/adolescent health
- Community service
- Mental health and well-being
- Personal empowerment/leadership
- Stress reduction (massage and yoga)
- Promoting healthy communities
- HIV/AIDS and STDs
- Accessing community resources
- Communication skills
- Complementary therapies

Also integrated into the course are activities for learning basic anatomy, including a review of the nervous, digestive, circulatory, reproductive, and respiratory systems.

Midway through the training course, participants are encouraged to become involved as volunteers in health promoter–directed projects at the center. In this way, we are able to identify potential leaders who will continue outreach to the community after completing the course. This intensive peer-to-peer approach requires that experienced health promoters provide extensive nurturing, encouragement, and mentoring of new health promoters.

PRIMARY HEALTH CARE INITIATIVES

The support from community institutions and the investment of time and energy into the health promoters training program has resulted in the development and successful implementation of eight community-based initiatives through Centro San Bonifacio. The health promoters function in various capacities and collaborate with other health services in multiple ways. They engage in assessing needs, organizing community health promotion activities (e.g., home visits, group education, individual risk-reduction education, health fairs, health-related campaigns, referrals to services), and work along side other healthcare providers and institutions to reduce access barriers. These initiatives include the following:

- *Multipliers Program.* This course provides baseline, intermediate, and advanced training on health promotion and disease prevention.
- *Community Food Pantry Anti-Hunger Project.* The food pantry provides supplemental food to needy families and the elderly through pantry membership. Also, the project provides hands-on organizing experience for local residents.
- *Provecto COMADRES ("Mother-to-Mother").* CHPs seek out pregnant women and provide prenatal education/intervention, home visiting, support, and referral; "doula" birth accompaniment (e.g., "servant" in Greek, and has traditionally been applied to women who provide labor support but who are not midwives); intensive breastfeeding promotion and support, and newborn care education and support; immunizations education and referrals, and infant safety seat promotion and distribution; and revitalization of the *cuarentena* tradition (40 days of postpartum rest and nurturing for mother and newborn). The CHPs actively advocate with healthcare providers and hospital staff to assure that clients have as little medical intervention as needed during birth, that breastfeeding can be initiated immediately after birth, and that babies are "roomed in" whenever possible. They are also strong advocates for access to a wide range of birth options for all women, including home births, free-standing birth centers, and access to midlevel providers such as certified nurse midwives.
- *Reducing Cultural Barriers to Health Care.* This project was a collaboration between Centro San Bonifacio, Erie Family Health Center, the Westside Health Authority, and the University of Illinois Midwest Latino Health Research, Policy, and Training Center. It consists of two major components: (1) a series of cross-cultural training workshops aimed at healthcare providers at Erie Family Health Center, which serves primarily Latino clients, and at Erie Westside, which serves primarily African Americans; (2) client orientations at the different sites on how to access and use the health center services, and on health topics and self-care skills in a number of health-related areas. In both components, CHPs play an integral role in the multidisciplinary team. The evaluation component, conducted by the University of Illinois at Chicago (UIC), assesses the impact of the cross-cultural workshops on Erie's healthcare providers. The evaluation also assessed the effectiveness of the CHP's interventions on patients in both communities, and the viability of the model in other settings.

Since the wrap up of this project, the effort has continued along serveral lines. At Erie Family Health Center, CHPs from Centro San Bonifacio continue to work on a number of community health education projects, especially with asthma prevention and breastfeeding promotion. At Centro San Bonifacio the CHPs are working in three areas:

- CHPs are collaborating with two groups in Latin America to organize an ongoing "Popular Medicine Academy" to train community residents on the appropriate use of medicinal plants, acupressure, and massage, as well as taking the workshops to other kinds of healthcare institutions such as universities, hospitals, and social services.

- CHPs are widening their outreach for provider training. They have developed two manuals: *Nuestra Cultura, Nuestra Salud: A Handbook on Latin American Health Beliefs and Practices* (Centro San Bonifacio, 1997a) and *Building Blocks to Better Health Care: A Multicultural Approach* (Centro San Bonifacio, 1997b). These manuals are disseminated nationally.

- In addition to educating the community about strategies to reduce violence, CHPs are using an individual, family, and community stress-reduction approach to violence prevention that incorporates massage, yoga, acupressure, exercise, plant-based therapies, and community education around domestic violence. Although still at the conceptual stage of development, CHPs are organizing a network of community safe houses in two community areas for women fleeing domestic violence. They accompany and advocate for women within the justice system and organize various individual, family, and community stress-reduction activities.

- *HIV/AIDS Prevention.* CHPs provide home-based education on HIV/AIDS and STD prevention, refer/follow-up for substance abuse treatment, HIV exams, and STD treatment. The program focuses on empowering families to communicate about HIV-related issues such as sexuality and risk behavior, helping individuals to reduce risk through condom use, effective communication and negotiation skills, substance abuse treatment, and mobilizing the community to engage in prevention activities.

- *Proyecto "San Cristobal."* A national network of sister communities working in solidarity with the Diocese of San Cristobal las Casas in Chiapas, Mexico. This project is building a network of support in the United States for bringing about social change and economic justice. It seeks to build support and solidarity for indigenous communities and self-development projects.

- *Leadership Development.* As a first step toward leadership development, Centro San Bonifacio encourages one-on-one informal counseling, peer support, encouragement, and nurturing for overcoming depression, resolving conflicts, professional development, and building self-esteem. After personal barriers are overcome, new CHPs participate in more advanced training including basic administration, protocols for meetings, appropriate professional dress, etc. As they assimilate and apply what they have learned, they are encouraged to participate in community boards and councils, assume more administrative responsibilities, and develop their own projects and initiatives. Moreover, CHPs actively seek collaborative relationships with individual professionals and organizations to facilitate their own ongoing training.

■ *Other Center Initiatives.* CHPs are encouraged to initiate and implement short- and long-term projects which they believe are needed in the community. For example, CHPs have presented several youth health promotion courses, a child health promoter training course using the Child-to-Child philosophy, a nutrition training project, and ongoing cardiopulmonary resuscitation and first aid training through the American Red Cross. Also, CHPs are encouraged to find their own training resources in the community and share these resources with other CHPs.

CENTRO SAN BONIFACIO: A PRIMARY HEALTH CARE MODEL

Effective primary health care (PHC) projects like Centro San Bonifacio are responsive to the sociocultural, economic, and political characteristics of a particular community, address the central health concerns and problems of the community, and provide access to promotive, preventive, curative, and rehabilitation services that address the health status and needs of the community. As mentioned in the introduction, Centro San Bonifacio was initiated by residents of an urban Hispanic/Latino community who understand the health beliefs and cultural values of the population they serve. Over the past six years the center has created many culturally relevant educational programs that teach individuals and families in their own neighborhoods to identify health problems and find solutions. In the spirit of "train-the-trainer" programs, the center trains CHPs who in turn provide a multitude of services: maternal child health promotion, illness prevention, ongoing CHP training, and health services such as the food dispensary, infant clothing exchange, healthcare referrals, and car seat distribution.

Centro San Bonifacio's model is effective because the CHPs live in the community where they work and share life experiences, values, and traditions. All of them begin as volunteers and because of their enthusiasm and the external moral and professional support they receive, they give much more than the work they are paid for in improving the health of their own neighborhoods. The CHPs personally reap the benefits of their investment as does the community at large.

Centro San Bonifacio promotes maximum community and individual self-reliance and participation in the planning, organization, operation, and control of each project. Trained health promoters are the backbone of the center. In the process of self-development, CHPs become skilled in working with other communities to build bridges to local service providers that effectively reduce cultural barriers. CHPs refer individuals and families to appropriate agencies, giving priority to needy families who have limited access to health services. By increasing their knowledge of local and national resources, CHPs have been effective community organizers. The result has been the development of culturally relevant approaches to healthcare.

Centro San Bonifacio relies on the support and collaboration of health professionals, including physicians, nurses, midwives, auxiliaries, and community workers, as well as traditional practitioners who are suitably trained with the social and technical skills necessary to complement the team. The center has an active advisory counsel composed of nurses, therapists, students, administrators, clergy, and CHPs. This group responds to the health needs of the community either through direct services or referrals, and assists the CHPs in all aspects of their professional development. As an institution, Centro San Bonifacio works closely with other local health promoter–driven agencies such as the Health Advocacy Project of Little Village and Centro Communitario Juan Diego.

KEY INSTITUTIONAL COLLABORATORS

The UIC has played an important role in supporting the development and legitimization of CHPs in Chicago since the late 1980s. The College of Nursing initiated one of the first training courses for community health advocates, and has provided this course specifically to empower community-based organizations that are looking to mobilize residents of their local areas for health promotion. They have also invited advanced health promoters to participate in their "Leadership for Primary Health Care" fellowship program, and have served as a fiscal agent for the Health Advocacy Project of Little Village, as well as placing their own health advocate in the West Town area through Erie Family Health Center. The Department of Emergency Medicine has facilitated a contract with the Illinois Department of Transportation to distribute car safety seats and provide related safety education through Centro San Bonifacio, the Health Advocacy Project of Little Village, and Centro Communitario "Juan Diego."

The UIC Jane Addams School of Social Work Latino Health Research, Policy, and Training Center has supported Centro San Bonifacio by conducting a two-year evaluation of its "Reducing Cultural Barriers to Health Care Project." Also, the UIC College of Nursing has lent its space for numerous events, including the annual Illinois health promoter conferences. In all, a broad, multifaceted, mutually respectful relationship between the community and the university has been developed. The uniqueness of this relationship lies in the fact that the emphasis has never been on finding subjects for research studies. On the contrary, UIC has lent technical assistance, support, and resources as a collaborator alongside the health promoters.

Several other large institutions have supported the development of Centro San Bonifacio's health promoters. The Latino Communities Area Health Education Center provides ongoing training and teaching assistance. Erie Family Health Center has given Centro San Bonifacio technical and moral support, as well as training since its inception. The Chicago Department of Public Health has also assisted with funding and program development, especially in the area of HIV/AIDS programing. The Illinois Institute of Technology Department of Rehabilitation Psychology has provided extensive training and assistance in evaluation methodologies for HIV/AIDS prevention. Many funding partners have made expansion of our programs possible.

DEVELOPING PHC NETWORKS

The PRO.ME.SA. Coalition was born out of a relationship established among three community-based, health promoter–driven organizations in Chicago: Centro San Bonifacio, Health Advocacy Project of Little Village (HAPLV), and Centro Communitario Juan Diego. The HAPLV, the oldest and most experienced of the three member agencies, was founded in 1990 with a strong affiliation to the UIC College of Nursing and the Chicago Department of Public Health. HAPLV uses a methodology based on reaching sectors of the neighborhood that are lacking in specific health services. Centro Communitario Juan Diego (CCJD), the newest of the three agencies, was founded in 1994 through the work of the Christian Base Communities. For several years previous to its founding, the members of the "Las Zelotas" community had been active in the South Chicago area with initiatives such as the United Neighborhood Organization and the local school councils. Through this process of trying to improve the circumstances around them, they decided to organize CCJD to foster leadership development and promote self-development within the Hispanic community.

"PRO.ME.SA.," which in Spanish means "promise," is derived from *Promotores y Promotoras por el Mejoramiento de la Salud*—"Promoters of Better Health." As health promoters from other community-based projects got to know one another, organized events together, and invited each other to training courses sponsored by the agencies, the CHPs began to realize that work could be consolidated and made more efficient if there were greater agency collaboration. The same principle also applied to fundraising and technical support for program development (in high demand among the three agencies). As the need to coordinate became more apparent, nine of the most experienced health promoters from the three organizations formed the board of directors for PRO.ME.SA. and began to organize the coalition.

The coalition maximizes the resources that are available to the Spanish-speaking communities of Chicago. The three agencies represented in PRO.ME.SA. have similar histories and methodologies; all focus on the training and mobilization of immigrant women as *promotoras* (health promoters) and have women at the forefront of their board, staff, and volunteer leadership. The board of directors is composed of 100 percent health promoters from the member agencies who are working in their neighborhoods. The uniqueness of this coalition is demonstrated by the fact that all member agencies are required to have boards of directors composed of at least 60 percent health promoters. This assures that the Coalition will remain a grassroots organization committed to supporting other grassroots organizations.

The coalition provides a forum for CHPs to share resources, develop methodologies with a common vision, and gain more public visibility. In addition to these functions, PRO.ME.SA. also organizes an annual statewide community health promoter conference (held each year at the UIC College of Nursing) where the CHPs can gain additional knowledge and skills in different, yet related, fields. Also at the annual conference, CHPs have an opportunity to present their own methodologies; a process that enables them to teach others, as well as gain input from other community-based organizations. During the conference, local CHPs are recognized for their activism and years of service in the community.

Coalition members share the belief that communities and individuals, if given the necessary tools, can organize for their own development and self-empowerment. Each member agency of the Coalition has developed its own health promoters training independently, although they have evolved in similar ways. One important element has been the collaboration from local health service providers in each area. Each agency has strong allies in the health service field and partners with various health providers and institutions in each community.

Health promoters from each agency are involved in advocacy activities at both the local and national level. Locally, CHPs advocate on a case-by-case basis on behalf of new immigrants who are trying to navigate the United States health system. As peers, the CHPs assist with finding services, making appointments, interpretation, conflict resolution with healthcare providers, and getting through much of the red tape of the health bureaucracy. This process involves becoming part of committees and other bodies that determine how health services are delivered. In addition, CHPs give testimony at citywide hearings, sit on several community boards and advisory groups, and serve as "cultural interpreters" for various community institutions, including local school councils, Chicago Department of Public Health clinic boards, and various community-based organizations and coalitions.

At the national level, the PRO.ME.SA. Coalition has participated in forums related to the role of the "community health worker." Through the New Professional section of the American Public Health Association, PRO.ME.SA. member agencies have participated in dialogue about defining and legitimizing the community health worker role, as well as obtaining credentials. Furthermore, the coalition has been part of the organizing committee for the national network of community health promoters. Centro San Bonifacio is represented in the planning group for this network which promotes mutual support among health promoters in different areas of the country. The network will provide an avenue for the interchange of ideas for developing successful community-based projects and strategies for accessing funding resources.

LESSONS LEARNED

One of the greatest lessons we have learned in this process of building a community-based organization is that creating true community ownership of the project must constantly be at the forefront of all activities. For the community to feel ownership of their work and successes, several factors must enter into the process.

- **Leadership Development**: The community, especially individuals involved in building the project, must have continual access to culturally and linguistically appropriate training on a myriad of subjects; "intermediate and advanced" training opportunities must also be accessible if participants are to grow. In addition to training, individuals should have opportunities to exercise the leadership they are developing—sitting on boards, advisory committees, acting as consultants, facilitating groups, coordinating projects, etc. Training and practice will eventually bring isolated community members into leadership positions.
- **Decision Making**: Participants must be the principal decision makers in the project. Community members need their own space to explore issues, discern direction, and gain assertiveness before real collaboration with professionals can take place. Often individuals may need time and encouragement before they feel comfortable to express their opinions and concerns openly and constructively. For this reason, Centro San Bonifacio maintained a board of directors composed of immigrant Hispanic community residents and a separate advisory council of professionals for four years before inviting professionals to join the board. Over time, the board gained sufficient autonomy and self-confidence to open 20 percent of its postions to the professional community.
- **Nurturing**: The community brings all its psychological, economic, social, and cultural dynamics into the organizing process. At varying levels, individuals may need a high level of attention to personal matters and the time to process life experiences before being able to function as organizers and promoters.
- **Participation**: Individuals should be able to participate in the projects or programs at many different levels, and the projects should be flexible enough to accommodate the different talents and skills of each person.
- **Informality**: The process of community organizing should be flexible enough to accommodate people with little formal education. For example, in organizing meetings there are value differences between professionals and community residents (i.e., professionals often place a high value on starting on time, whereas the community may pay less attention to the clock than to the arrival of key people).
- **Geography**: Having a place to call "our own" is extremely important in claiming our own identity as opposed to being located in an office of a larger institution such as a university or hospital. Currently our office is located in the community we serve in a free-standing public housing unit loaned by the Illinois Lutheran Social Services.
- **Community Building**: Centro San Bonifacio was born out of crisis when the St. Bonifacio parish closed. A cluster of families involved in the community conceived the idea of developing the center primarily as a means to sustain the community life of the parish. For the first several years the center served this purpose; however, crisis-response organizing cannot sustain itself. The center realized that rather than continue to reflect on the trauma of the past we needed to look to the future and develop our programs accordingly.

CONCLUSION

Over the past five years that we have been working in the area of health promotion, our main focus has been the training and mobilization of community health promoters. Our collective process of self-empowerment, raising awareness (both personal and community), leadership development, and community involvement has been challenging and gratifying. Like other PHC models (McFarland, 1996), our efforts to bring public, private, and political sectors of the community together has centered on empowerment through unity, training women and men as effective health promoters, and the shared belief that community residents are capable of identifying and meeting their own health needs. This continues to be Centro San Bonifacio's vision for the future.

REFERENCES

Centro San Bonifacio. (1997a). *Nuestra cultura, nuestra salud: A handbook on Latin American health beliefs and practices.* Chicago, IL: Centro San Bonifacio.

Centro San Bonifacio. (1997b). *Building blocks for better health care: A multicultural approach.* Chicago, IL: Centro San Bonifacio.

Chicago Department of Public Health. (November, 1995). *An epidemiologic profile of HIV/AIDS in Chicago.*

Council on Scientific Affairs. (1991). Hispanic health in the United States. *Journal of the American Medical Association, 265,* 248–252.

Diaz, T., Buehler, J., Castro, K., & Ward, J. (1993). AIDS trends among Hispanics in the United States. *American Journal of Public Health, 83*(4), 504–509.

McFarland, J. (1996). De Madres a Madres: An access model for primary care. *American Journal of Public Health, 86*(6), 879–880.

Novello, A., Wise, P., & Kleiman, D. (1991). Hispanic health: Time for data, time for action. *Journal of the American Medical Association, 26,*(2), 253–255.

Chapter 13

Chicago Health Connection: Developing Community Leadership in Maternal and Child Health

RACHEL ABRAMSON
JERETHA MCKINLEY

Acknowledgments:
The authors extend grateful recognition to the Chicago Health Connection team (past and present). Tamara Adams, Rossana Barrera, Bertha Condes, Helen Dimas, Peg Dublin, Pamela King, Regina Pitts, and Judy Teibloom-Mishkin. We are indebted to the hundreds of peer counselors who have taught us the most essential truths and have given the best of themselves to their communities. Finally, we gratefully acknowledge the help of our board of directors, our supporters and our funders, including Best Start, Inc., the Boston Foundation, the Chicago Community Trust, the Chicago Foundation for Women, the Cook County Hospital Auxiliary, the Cook County Hospital Perinatal Center, A Girl's Best Friend Foundation, the Harris Foundation, the Illinois Department of Public Health, the Ounce of Prevention Fund, the Pittway Corporation, the Polk Bros. Foundation, the Robert Wood Johnson Foundation, the Seabury Foundation, the Otho S. A. Sprague Memorial Institute, the University of Chicago Graduate School of Business, and the U.S. Committee for UNICEF.

It was through a process of engagement with natural leaders in a variety of communities that Chicago Health Connection (CHC) expanded a grassroots approach to breastfeeding promotion into a model program for community-based maternal and child health promotion. Formerly the Chicago Breastfeeding Task Force, CHC is dedicated to promoting the health and well-being of low-income mothers, their young children and families. CHC uses peer counseling, training, support, research, and advocacy to enhance the capacity of low-income women to address their heathcare needs. Since 1986, CHC has trained more than 650 low-income mothers and thousands of professional and lay health workers who serve within their own neighborhoods by promoting breastfeeding, infant immunizations, birthing support, and other health promotion strategies.

ORGANIZATIONAL HISTORY

CHC's work has come to include a characteristically open, respectful approach to supporting community and institutional efforts to define and address healthcare needs. However, our initial work was much more narrowly defined. The Chicago Breastfeeding Task Force was formed in 1986 as a coalition of healthcare providers and consumers who were interested in promoting breastfeeding in low-income communities as an infant mortality reduction strategy. All of the participants were passionate about breastfeeding, and aware of the challenges and personal frustration involved in promoting a practice that was not the cultural norm in many communities. Our personal experiences, informed by our knowledge of other community-based efforts, determined the direction of our work. By 1987, our agency began doing peer counselor training and placement in breastfeeding promotion as a response to personal experiences as healthcare providers and consumers with the failure of traditional information-based prevention strategies.

The first Breastfeeding Peer Counselor Project, based on a community lay worker model, was established as a pilot project at Cook County Hospital. After a year of organizational assessment and staff development, we initiated the first breastfeeding peer counselor training. Sessions covered basic breastfeeding promotion issues and management techniques, and quickly expanded to a twenty-hour course, which included counseling techniques, parenting, infant development, and other topics in maternal and infant health promotion. The first cadre of trained peer counselors began supporting breastfeeding mothers in 1987. By recruiting trainees from the postpartum wards, within five years, breastfeeding rates at Cook County Hospital had increased from 21 percent to 50 percent.

The successful institutionalization of that program (it continues today as a joint program of the Cook County Hospital Perinatal Center and CHC) allowed CHC to expand the pilot. Since then, we have established similar programs in a number of hospitals and clinics, and have worked extensively with the Illinois Women, Infants and Children (WIC) program. Very early in our history it became clear that the power of the program rested with the community women who worked as peer counselors. Their experiences and their issues directed the subsequent development of the organization.

The success of the peer counselor work has been based on a model that identifies successful natural leaders, and then "nurtures the nurturers." Successful breastfeeding is an empowering experience for a woman. Peer counselor training supports and confirms a woman's strengths and gives her a sense of her own internal power to help others to have the same experience. Similarly, when community health advocates feel successful in meeting their own needs, they are then able to teach others the same self-care practices.

Early in the development of the CHC, we found that when peer counselors established a supportive, trusted relationship with their clients, they became not only a source of information and nurturing, but also the critical link to healthcare and social services. When there was a problem in the family of any sort, it was the peer counselor who was asked for help. The counselors were constantly asking for more training in other areas of maternal-child health and family support. We came to see breastfeeding as a window into women's lives at a time of great need and great openness. Hence, over time the focus of the program shifted from breastfeeding as an infant health strategy to a broader, more holistic model of community-based maternal support.

CHC works with community members and professional staff of health and social service agencies to develop health promotion approaches around health issues identified by the community and the agency. Training and consultation are based on principles of "empowerment education," developed by Brazilian educator Paulo Freire; "imaginal learning," developed by Kenneth Boulding (1956) and expanded by the Chicago-based Institute for Cultural Affairs (Seagren, 1988); and on a respectful process of listening to natural community leaders and facilitating grassroots advocacy efforts.

Empowerment education is a dynamic and effective model of health education and community development focusing on personal and social change. The model is based on the philosophy of Paulo Freire (1970), a successful Brazilian educator, who transformed objects and pictures into culturally potent symbols in order to challenge students to think critically about their lives and to learn how to control their destinies. The principle of dialogue is basic to this methodology. All of the participants (both teachers and students) are considered integral to a learning process that is mutually informing.

At CHC, Freirian principles of education and community development undergird our philosophical approach to building healthy communities. CHC training sessions are highly interactive, drawing from participants' life experiences. Curricula are developed in collaboration with culturally diverse members of the community. Often peer counselors are included as members of the training team to share their valuable perspective with participants. The goal is to achieve an active process of learning that results in a change in the way participants view the world and their role as change agents.

Imaginal earning postulates that people behave according to their image of the reality of the world. If we believe that true learning occurs as we change from an old mind-set (also called image or paradigm) to a new mind-set, we must base our training activities on what we believe to be the old image held by the participants. The old image directs people's behavior until they discover how it doesn't work (or develop a more complex understanding of how it does work). The activities and information experienced by the participants challenges the old mind set and allows the formation of a new mind-set informed by new knowledge and new experience.

Assessing the mind-set of an audience is a difficult skill to learn. The best way to discover the deepest feelings of a group is simply to listen over a period of time to what concerns people most. The issues that generate strong emotions and energy in a community are those that will motivate people to learn and act toward change.

Focusing on this process of discovery and change in small groups and larger communities has stimulated our organizational development. CHC has moved from a single-issue task force to an independent agency which supports and develops community-based leadership in broad areas of maternal and child health promotion.

In 1993, incorporating elements of Freirian training, imaginal learning, and community organizing, CHC began to expand its work to other areas of maternal-child health promotion, including immunization promotion, lead prevention, asthma support, and support for birthing teens. As with some life-cycle events, the change in our situation was marked by a new name. In 1995, we transitioned from our old status as the Chicago Breastfeeding Task Force, and became Chicago Health Connection, an independent nonprofit corporation with a broader mission in health promotion and support. Our decision to expand the program into community-based advocacy and birthing support was confirmed by the enthusiasm of the community and the success of our projects.

After a number of years of learning from both successful and unsuccessful projects, CHC moved into training healthcare professionals and paraprofessionals to effectively utilize this model to better serve low-income communities. We were asked to provide more training and consultation to agencies and institutions who were interested in developing programs using the peer counselor role. CHC now conducts three-day training conferences both locally and in other cities that are attended by participants from all over the country.

Our local grassroots work continues to be the heart of our program. Any knowledge or expertise we have gained is drawn directly from the many women who work tirelessly to support other women in making healthy choices in their lives and in the lives of their children.

A PROCESS OF DISCOVERY

We have never ceased to be impressed with the power of peer counselors' support and leadership for health in their communities. Program evaluations have shown dramatic increases in health outcomes after peer counselor programs were instituted in hospitals or clinics. A study of the program at Cook County

Hospital showed significant differences in rates of breastfeeding initiation, duration, and exclusivity for women who had peer counselor support. At Lawndale Christian Health Center, breastfeeding rates increased from 21 percent to 61 percent within three months of placement of a Spanish-speaking peer counselor. In the first year of an intensive community-based birthing support project for teens (the Chicago Health Connection Doula Project), the Caesarian section rate was less than half of the national average for adolescents, and the breastfeeding initiation rate was 84 percent. We estimate that each month peer counselors in Illinois contact a total of 14,000 low-income pregnant or breastfeeding women.

We have also been struck with the changes that develop in the lives of the women who assume the peer counselor role. We have watched peer counselors move forward with educational plans, obtain their first paying jobs, buy property, share child care, and start businesses. We are convinced of the importance of the peer counselor role, both in health promotion, and in individual and community development. Besides providing an effective model for supporting healthy choices for women and their children and increasing access to the healthcare system, this role seems to be transformational for women who have not necessarily had other successes in their lives. Once they experience their power to help other women, they seem to be ready to take powerful steps in their lives, including the first steps toward economic self-sufficiency.

What we have learned from the peer counselors has affected every aspect of our work. Observing the profound personal and community changes brought about by this approach, and the strength of the resources within communities, we are constantly challenged to reshape, improve, and push forward. As peer counselors transform their own lives, they also push CHC to grapple with the complicated process of facilitating community-based change around maternal and child health issues.

The culture of our organization supports a continual expansion of vision and a dynamic response to both political and experiential events. CHC bases much of its approach to community health on the essential process of critical self-examination through program evaluation. We value our successes but we consider what we learn when programs don't work as we have planned them just as valuable. Usually, we find that if clients or communities aren't participating in a project it is because we have made incorrect assumptions and tried to impose our own predetermined goals on the community.

The principles of Freirian training emphasize listening and responding to the community's concerns. To be successful in harnessing this powerful resource, we are constantly learning more about how to give community members the opportunity to connect the personal with the theoretical, and to think critically about the problems, resources, and potential solutions in their midst. CHC is experienced in planning and conducting events that allow this process to happen. Whenever we have done so, we have seen the motivation and action planning that it takes for a community to take on a problem in a real way.

LIVING ON THE EDGE

Because CHC's program is not geographically concentrated and does not operate out of a single health or social service institution, we have always relied on intersectoral collaboration. This circumstance has both sharpened our listening skills and trust-building abilities and heightened the challenges of sustaining primary health care (PHC) programs. As we work with institutions to develop and support peer counselor projects, we are struck with how powerful, challenging, and risky this model can be.

When we enter into a partnership with community members for the purpose of improving community health, we make a commitment to begin a journey into unknown territory. True partnership involves both respect for differences and the ability to come to a common purpose. In training and placing breastfeeding peer counselors, CHC had to learn to listen to the priorities of the counselors, both in how they wanted to learn and what they needed to learn. As we broadened our focus, we were forced to pay attention to our own assumptions and the needs of the communities in which we were working. As we approached groups of natural leaders, we would ask them, "What are the things that you would like to address when it comes to children's health and particularly as it has to do with breastfeeding?" Our challenge was to develop the courage and ability to support those communities when their priorities were different from what we had assumed.

Community members have told us by their lack of involvement in a project that we had not tapped their critical issues. They did not "own" the project as we had initially conceived it. We learned that if we respect them, then we must give them an opportunity to tell us about their health issues and concerns. If we listen, we can gather the resources necessary to act on their vision.

We continue to be challenged by the need to convince funders and provider agencies to allow the change process to take place as the communities define their own needs and priorities. We walk a fine line when we approach institutions and ask to partner with them on a project. Communicating our perceptions of the needs of the community has to be balanced with respect and acknowledgment of what the institution values and is willing to offer.

Successfully integrating lay community health workers into agencies also requires a serious process of preparing both the worker and the agency. Relying on lay people to provide "services" is a big change for some healthcare providers who are comfortable with thinking of community people as "consumers," or receivers of needed services. The scope and limitations of the peer counselor's role, which is not a traditional role, need to be understood and seen as valuable by all the "stakeholders" in an agency. CHC has developed extensive community and institutional contacts throughout the Chicago area and approaches the marketing of this model as a community-organizing exercise, requiring respectful engagement with all levels of potential support for and resistance to the model. Issues of training, support, and supervision of women who may not have been in the work force prior to their involvement in the project become critical for the success of a project.

CHC is moving toward program expansion in two areas. We are increasingly engaged in our role as an independent training and consulting agency with other agencies interested in instituting community-based maternal-child health promotion programs. Our reputation has grown throughout the city, along with far-reaching networks that encompass a variety of people working with low-income women. Simultaneously, our expanding Peer Counselor Network provides compensation for the peer counselors' work, opportunities for continuing education and professional development, newsletter development, speaking engagements, employment preparation, and the nurturing and support that women need to continue to nurture others. We are in contact with more than 200 of the 600 peer counselors we have trained. They have the potential to affect the lives of thousands of other women. Their work exemplifies the PHC model and their experience continues to drive CHC's development.

LESSONS LEARNED

We learned, first of all, that a PHC model is both powerful and fragile. We found over time that in spite of excellent skills in connecting with and supporting their clients, peer counselors and their agencies needed more supervision and support than we had initially expected and budgeted for. We are consistently faced with this issue, but often are still under-budget for peer counselor supervision and support, because of the funder's priorities. It is a challenge to find ways to communicate to funders and administrators that this kind of program is not a "cheap" program, even though the average compensation levels for peer counselors are relatively (and regrettably) low. PHC programs are highly effective, but can be complicated to develop and implement. It is critical that they be marketed on the basis of their effectiveness with a full and upfront understanding of the resources necessary for success.

Secondly, we learned through this work that we will not have sustainable, long-term success with a new initiative unless we involve all stakeholders at the onset of planning of the program. "Listening to our audiences" is crucial to establishing access and to developing the most appropriate strategic and programmatic directions for a particular setting. Particularly in our role as an independent collaborating or consulting agency, CHC has to be clear about involving stakeholders from every level of a community, respecting the opinions of staff and administration as much as those of community members most affected by the issues being addressed.

We learned that real change takes time. In some communities in which we worked it took four or five years for a project to really take hold. This reality is an expensive endeavor. In the past, the expense was often borne by our agency because we continued to work with selected communities long after the traditional one or two years of funding ran out. Hence we are now bolder in asking funders and agency providers to partner with us in committing the resources that it takes to enable communities to address their critical health issues. Community-based health promotion will not be successful unless it is driven by a collaborative process, in which the community's many voices are clearly heard. As CHC matures, we are becoming more successful in broadening our sources of financial support and in communicating the actual costs of collaborative change.

The CHC's organization and programs are rooted in its community work. We feel fortunate to be engaged in supporting the kind of critical process that enables important changes to take place. As an organization and as individuals, we also reap the benefits of lessons learned, allies made, and the inspiration and energy that flows from the work of personal and community transformation.

REFERENCES

Boulding, K. (1956). *The image: Knowledge in life and society.* Ann Arbor: University of Michigan Press.
Freire, P. (1970). *Pedagogy of the oppressed.* New York: Seabury Press.
Seagren, R. (1988). Imaginal education. *In Context, 18,* 58–51.

Chapter 14

Peer Education for AIDS Prevention in Multiethnic Non-English-Speaking Communities

MAYUMI ANNE WILLGERODT
CAROL CHRISTIANSEN
JOANNA SU

The authors gratefully acknowledge the editorial assistance of Randy Spreen Parker and Kathleen Norr in the preparation of this chapter. We would also like to thank all of the participating women in the Uptown community for their dedication and work in improving the health of their community.

INTRODUCTION

Primary health care (PHC) examines health in the context of community, and can be used as a model for developing, implementing, and evaluating health promotion initiatives. The PHC model is particularly effective for multiethnic minority communities because it recognizes the social and economic processes that impact health status. This chapter describes an HIV/AIDS education program implemented as part of a larger health education project in five ethnic communities and identifies issues for consideration when planning health promotion programs.

History

The Mutual Aid Associations' (MAA) Women's Health Education Project (MWHEP) is a collaborative effort of five not-for-profit MAAs-social service agencies which were founded by and for refugee and immigrant communities. The five MAAs—the Cambodian Association of Illinois, Chinese Mutual Aid Association, Ethiopian Community Association of Chicago, Lao-American Community Services, and the Vietnamese Association of Illinois—were all established in the mid-1970s to early 80s. They are located in the Uptown community area, which has historically been Chicago's point of entry for numerous immigrant and refugee groups. Because these organizations have similar missions and services, and their communities share common challenges and struggles, the MAAs have worked together on a number of projects over the last decade. Building collaborative relationships and sharing resources has strengthened these programs.

The MWHEP, one of several current joint MAA ventures, was established in 1994 through a United Way Health Priority Grant, grants from the U.S. Office of Minority Health, and the Johnson & Johnson Community Health Care Program, support from the Chicago Foundation for Women. Currently, the project is funded primarily by the United Way and the Illinois Department of Public Health. The goal of MWHEP is to increase access to and understanding of preventive and PHC among low-income, limited English-speaking refugee and immigrant women. The project targets women who, as the traditional caretakers of the family, can influence healthcare decisions. The health of families and communities can be improved by reaching out to women.

The strategies to increase health access and awareness focus on developing bilingual, bicultural health resources in the five communities. Culturally appropriate, multilingual resource materials have been developed and community health advocate staff and volunteer peer health educators are utilized to improve the health of the communities. In addition to these direct service strategies, project staff also work with area hospitals, clinics, and health networks to improve healthcare service delivery to refugee and immigrant populations.

Much of the MWHEP's effectiveness can be attributed to the structure of the program; the project's lead agency is an MAA with direct ties to and experience with the target population. In addition to having a full-time bicultural project coordinator at the Vietnamese Association, each of the MAAs has a full-time bilingual, bicultural female health advocate staff who has received training from healthcare and social service professionals on numerous healthcare topics, including tuberculosis, hepatitis, breast cancer, cervical cancer, hypertension, HIV/AIDS, domestic violence, child abuse, and prenatal care. All of the health advocates themselves are refugees or immigrants, and have firsthand experience with the challenges of adjusting to a new country.

These trained health advocates provide direct services in the community to women. These services include health education (in one-to-one as well as small group settings) and mediation between healthcare providers/systems and community members with limited English proficiency. In addition, a key component of MWHEP is peer education. Through interactions with community members and discussions with community leaders, health advocates have identified and recruited community women to become prepared as peer health educators, targeting women who are active in their communities, enjoy talking and sharing with others, and have a desire to help their communities.

In the spring of 1995, the first series of peer health educator training sessions was held and included discussions of Western versus home country health beliefs and practices, nutrition and diet, women's health screenings, hypertension, and prenatal care. As part of a continuing community research project directed by faculty and staff of a local academic institution, a module focusing on breast cancer education has also been implemented.

An HIV/AIDS prevention education module was developed out of an interest expressed by the five communities and students and faculty at the University of Illinois at Chicago (UIC), College of Nursing. The UIC staff had firsthand experience with HIV/AIDS prevention education and the concept of peer education from a program implemented in Botswana, South Africa (Norr et al., 1992). Because the program was successful and many of the principles and underlying issues related to women and HIV are similar, the Botswana project was used as the model for the Chicago program.

BACKGROUND

The success of the HIV/AIDS peer education prevention program in Botswana demonstrated conclusively that educating community women is essential to contain the spread of HIV infection. In their key roles as healthcare decision makers and educators within the family and the community, women consistently proved their ability to have impact on the health of the community (Norr et al., 1992). Providing women with accurate information on HIV/AIDS has the potential to positively influence the health-related behaviors of families and communities. These facts, as well as the knowledge and understanding gained from the Botswana experience, provided the initial impetus and direction for the pilot project in Chicago with the five communities that were a part of the MWHEP. Utilizing a community-based PHC approach, this project attempted to build on the strengths of the existing social

networks previously established within each community by the health advocates and peer educators vis-à-vis the MWHEP. Program leaders anticipated
that the use of a social learning model in peer-led groups would enable women
to affect attitudinal and behavioral changes that would eventually lead to a
reduction in HIV/AIDS risk behaviors. The peer education training manual is
available on request from the UIC World Health Organizations Collaborating
Center.

The concept of peer education is congruent with the PHC model in that
peer education actively promotes self-care and self-reliance (Norr et al., 1992).
Also, the model is especially amenable to HIV/AIDS prevention. This is
because it is based on the recognition that behaviors are part of complex social
patterns that involve not only the individual, but also entire social networks and
value systems. Thus, the peer education model provides ongoing support for
the individual as well as the group when long-standing ways of thinking and
behaving are challenged. The peer education model fosters the development of
new patterns of behavior.

The project trains volunteers to be group leaders. Once trained, group
leaders organize and conduct groups of their own in communities, schools,
churches, or the workplace. Ideally, group leaders are linked to a community-
based nurse or other health professional that provides ongoing consultation
and expertise for training, support for peer group leaders, and coordination of
project expansion.

In this project, each of the peer groups in the five communities was
supervised by the trained community health advocates (CHAs) who were
employed staff members of their respective MAAs. In general, the CHAs demonstrated better language skills, and were more educated and assimilated than
the peer educators under their supervision. In each of the communities, the
CHAs had a close working relationship with the peer educators and assisted
them in the direction of their work with families and individuals. Because of
their key positions within the MAA, and their close working relationships with
the peer educators, the CHAs were crucial to the success of the MWHEP
project as well as the HIV/AIDS prevention project. During the planning and
implementation stages of this project, the CHAs worked closely with the
project staff in reviewing course content and materials and in offering continuous feedback.

ISSUES ENCOUNTERED:
PROGRAM PLANNING
AND COURSE CONTENT

The program was structured so that over a period of seven or more sessions,
women would gain confidence in their knowledge and understanding of sexually transmitted diseases (STDs), especially HIV/AIDS. The curriculum also
prepared women to identify the practices and behaviors that increased their
risk of contracting HIV/AIDS or other STDs. The lessons were prepared

consecutively, following a logical sequence and building one upon the other. The materials were presented in such a way that they could easily be tailored to meet specific cultural expectations and requirements. Because a modular approach was used in developing the teaching materials, the order of presentation could also be readily altered to fit the needs of the group.

The project staff planned to follow the original model, presenting the material in seven sessions. In the planning stages, the CHAs from each of the five communities, the project coordinator of MWHEP, and instructors from the UIC coordinated the program logistics. All the CHAs agreed that the peer educators would demonstrate a higher degree of cooperation and interest if the material was condensed and presented in a shorter time period. Subsequently, in each of the communities the course was offered in four weeks. The majority of the classes were held on Saturdays beginning in mid-January of 1996.

Changing the format and condensing the course proved to be problematic for the program staff, posing several problems. First, when peer educators were absent or late due to family concerns or weather conditions, the group was too small for the dynamic interplay that is necessary for group work. Second, arranging make-up sessions was difficult. It became the responsibility of the CHAs to meet individually with the peer educators who had missed sessions to review the teaching content. This created issues of quality control for the staff. Because the teaching methods were dependent on group dynamics and discussion, how closely the make-up sessions approximated the material covered in the classes is unclear.

Language barriers posed an additional challenge in disseminating the HIV/AIDS prevention message. Since most peer educators are not bilingual, the classes were simultaneously translated by the CHAs into their respective languages. There was difficulty in ensuring that technical, health-related information was transmitted correctly and consistently by the CHAs during the classes. Also, having peer educators who were not bilingual restricted their ability to bridge the English-speaking healthcare system for their clients.

Early in the program, almost an entire session was devoted to a review of male and female anatomy and physiology. As a part of this session, the instructors listed the proper names of each of the body parts concerned with sexual functioning. The group was then asked to give all the names (including slang terms) used by their culture for the same parts of the body. Then, as a group, the peer educators were asked to decide on the terms they believed to be appropriate for use when teaching in the community. The purpose of this exercise was to clarify the fact that each culture uses numerous terms to describe the body and that personal embarrassment in utilizing some of these terms can interfere with clear communication. Group consensus in choosing terms was meant to minimize the discomfort peer educators experienced with certain terms, and to ensure the cultural appropriateness of terms selected for use. Given the sensitive nature of the topic, this exercise proved to be beneficial in reducing the tension and discomfort initially experienced by group members as these topics were introduced.

Another session was devoted to the correct use of condoms. In this session, participants were given condoms in class and taught the proper way of removing the condom from its wrapper and the appropriate techniques for condom care, use, and disposal. For demonstration purposes, the use of an anatomical model made of synthetic material was recommended when practicing the correct use of condom application. This technique for demonstrating condom use proved to be inappropriate for the peer educators who expressed uneasiness with this method. Instead, groups chose to use their hands as demonstration models for condom application. The peer educators also stated that they would be reluctant to demonstrate condom use to community women outside of the classroom setting. Social and cultural barriers of this nature proved to be significant factors that limited the growth of the program within these communities.

The program made liberal use of group discussions and activities such as role play. The role play was designed to assist women in decision making and in developing the negotiation skills needed for practicing safer sex. The program manual suggested different scenarios for the role play, each presenting somewhat difficult situations women might encounter with new or existing sexual partners.

In these situations, within the security of the group, women were presented with the opportunity to begin dialogue with their partners concerning sexuality and safe sex practices. This activity was difficult for the peer educators because for the most part, it represented the first time that they openly discussed issues of a sexual nature in this way. Role playing also required "confronting" one's partner, which was not consistent with the cultural norms of these communities. For this reason, many of the women chose not to participate. Because the instructors and CHAs felt that role play was a crucial component of learning, the peer educators were asked to identify scenarios that were more realistic and feasible in their culture. These scenarios were used for the remainder of the lessons.

PEER EDUCATORS AND THE COMMUNITY

Although the peer educators completed the training, they had a great deal of difficulty with the sexually explicit content of the program and with the exercises that dealt with partner negotiations. They acknowledged to the instructors and CHAs that the interventions that they would bring to the community would most likely occur on a one-to-one basis rather in groups. The staff reasoned that because most of the peer educators were mature women, probably not at high personal risk, they may have thought it inappropriate or unnecessary to discuss these issues with women who were their contemporaries. Additionally, in the cultures represented by these communities, it is considered inappropriate to discuss sexual issues across generational lines. This made it difficult for many of the peer educators to have open discussions with younger women who may have been in higher risk categories. Also, the CHAs may have overestimated the peer educators' willingness to take on the issue of HIV/

AIDS. Because of age, social status, and language limitations, the peer educators who were in place at the time the program was initiated were probably not the most appropriate for this task.

The staff also concluded at the completion of the program that because HIV/AIDS was not widespread in these communities, the peer educators may have been more interested in obtaining factual information about the disease and less interested in becoming involved in a larger prevention program. It is also possible that while there may have been genuine interest in the topic, other issues were of greater priority. Throughout the program, however, women were encouraged to develop a plan for personal safety . . . one that included abstinence from sexual relations among unmarried women, and/or the appropriate use of condoms, and recognition that women are potentially at risk due to their partners' behaviors as well as their own. The program assisted in improving the leadership skills and the communication skills of the participants.

DISCUSSION

The HIV/AIDS prevention program involved initial pilot work with an urban immigrant women's group with which we had no prior experience. Most of our previous efforts in PHC had focused on other ethnic communities with cultural values, norms, and behaviors that differed from the five communities with whom we worked. In light of the issues that have been raised in our program, several recommendations for the implementation of future community programs are outlined below.

PEER EDUCATORS IN RELATION TO THE PROGRAM CONTENT

The literature indicates that the selection of peer educators is crucial to the success of community-based health promotion programs (Norr et al., & Tlou, 1992; Swider & McElmurry, 1990). Peer educators must be leaders in the community with a sense of vision and dedication. In addition, the HIV/AIDS program required that people be at ease with issues surrounding sexuality. The women who were selected for this program had not yet developed the skills necessary to educate the community about HIV/AIDS. Although these women demonstrated the requisite leadership, vision, and dedication, their uneasiness with sexual issues limited their effectiveness and posed unexpected challenges to the implementation of the project. Thus, HIV/AIDS prevention, and potentially other types of health promotion, has requirements beyond those usually identified as important for peer educators.

The general consensus of the instructors was that the peer educators were not unlike other women in the community, who were also unlikely to feel comfortable discussing sexuality. The instructors recognized that unless the peer educators developed comfort in discussing sexuality, they would be ineffective at conveying the information to the community. Therefore, the instructors decided to focus the lessons on assisting the women to talk about sexuality and meeting the needs of the women. Given the comfort level of the peer educators, the instructors identified and prioritized the essential HIV/AIDS prevention information. This information was then conveyed to the community.

Selection of appropriate peer educators is crucial to the successful implementation of a health education program. Peer educators must not only be dedicated leaders with the time to educate communities, but they must also be comfortable with the content of their "message." In this sense, focus groups or informal meetings with representatives from the community should be conducted throughout the planning process to get a sense of the community and determine the level of comfort in relation to the program content. Peer educators may be selected based on who the target audience is, who the leaders in the targeted audience are, and who is comfortable with the content. This type of assessment should be conducted with *each* program so that the best "fit" between peer educator and program may be achieved.

As previously noted, the personal values and belief systems of the peer educators were a barrier in disseminating HIV/AIDS information. The peer educators did not feel that the women in the community they would be targeting were truly at risk for HIV. They believed that the threat of HIV and AIDS was restricted to homosexuals and intravenous drug users. Over time however, the instructors were successful in convincing the peer educators that the most effective HIV/AIDS prevention requires that all members of the community, regardless of age, marital status, or sexual orientation, be willing to discuss sexual issues openly. The differences in views between the instructors and the peer educators on who is at risk for HIV underscore the need to clearly identify mutual goals at the onset of any program and to evaluate these goals throughout the course of the program. Differences in the perceived severity of and susceptibility to the problem must be resolved for any collaborative community program to be successful. Furthermore, all participants must agree on the process by which the goals are to be achieved.

THE COMMUNITY IN RELATION TO THE PROGRAM

The feasibility of implementing a program must be established in a way that meets the needs of a given community. Careful consideration must be given to availability of resources and time investment. All too often, health promotion programs are implemented in a community without adequate knowledge of the time, financial requirements, and commitment of personnel that is needed and as a result, many community interventions do not adequately educate the community and comprehensively promote health. When the appropriate resources are lacking, decisions need to be made on the feasibility and eventual success of the proposed program. This means that (at times) programs should not be initiated until a more appropriate time when those commitments may be made. This decision is balanced by the need to capitalize on the community's readiness and interest in implementing a health education program.

Program evaluation is necessary in order to determine the outcome of a program. However, many community programs either are not evaluated until the conclusion of a program or do not include participant feedback. As a result, any valuable lessons that are learned cannot be initiated until a new program is developed. This is disappointing in that the opportunity to make adjustments in a particular program to better meet the needs of a community has been lost. Community-based programs should develop an evaluation plan that allows for assessments by the participants throughout the program. Time should be factored in the program to reflect on its process so that any changes that need to occur to ensure its success can be made during the program.

The HIV/AIDS peer education prevention program yielded several positive outcomes for the community and the instructors. First, the program provided the opportunity to introduce the topic of HIV/AIDS into the community. Dialogue about sexuality and STDs was initiated which, in turn, allowed the women to discuss relationships between men and women, including gender and power inequalities, the threat of violence, and negotiation skills to use with partners. Second, the manual for HIV/AIDS prevention education was revised to be more flexible to accommodate different communities. Brief summary cards were developed for distribution that summarize AIDS facts and display proper condom usage in the five respective languages. Last, the program also forged ties between the five ethnic communities and utilized the UIC at Chicago as a resource for technical assistance. The communities and the UIC continue to work together in identifying how to best serve the community and promote health. In addition, the UIC placed a graduate student intern in these communities.

The cultural and language issues encountered were unanticipated challenges in the implementation of this program. In particular, the cultural barriers surrounding discussion of sexual risks of HIV/AIDS transmission were underestimated, in part reflecting the greater acculturation of leaders than community women. In the future, a longer program with more general PHC activities (such as overall women's health) initially might develop the trust and comfort needed to deal with more sensitive topics. The instructors learned a great deal about their own assumptions about the ability to confront sexuality issues, and the teaching of sensitive health information.

Despite the challenges and issues encountered in this program, this experience provided a unique learning opportunity for the project staff. Adequate program planning not only includes coordinating the logistics of a program, but also assessing the community's "readiness" for the content of the program. Peer educators must be evaluated for appropriateness for each type of program in order to ensure accurate and appropriate dissemination of health information. Finally, community programs must be flexible and amenable to modification as the needs of a community become evident over time.

CONCLUSION

PHC addresses health in the context of availability, accessibility, and affordability of services and is inextricably linked to social and economic processes within a community. Without consideration of issues such as equity and community participation, Health for All cannot be achieved (World Health Organization, 1978). The issues that were raised in this chapter illustrate the importance of community involvement for successful health promotion programs. Working with communities and planning the programs is a process that requires engagement and commitment. To ensure a successful program, planning must not only include determining appropriate content, but also exploring community readiness, establishing mutual goals for process and outcomes, and assessing feasibility. PHC provides a framework to facilitate this process.

References

Norr, K. F., McElmurry, B. J., Moeti, M., & Tlou, S. D. (1994). AIDS prevention for women: A community-based approach. In S. J. Ouerberg (Ed.), *AIDS, ethics and religion* (pp.189–199). New York: Orbis Books.

Norr, K. F., McElmurry, B. J., Moeti, M., & Tlou, S. D. (1992). AIDS prevention for women: A community-based approach. *Nursing Outlook, 40*(6), 250–256.

Norr, K. F., McElmurry, B. J., & Tlou, S. D. (1997). *Women and HIV/AIDS prevention: A global approach. Peer education program: Training manual.* Chicago: WHO Collaborating Center.

World Health Organization. (1978). *Primary health care.* Geneva: World Health Organization.

Chapter 15

Primary Health Care for Urban School Children: Developing Comprehensive School Health Programs for Inner-City Children

B. JOAN NEWCOMB

Acknowledgments:

I would like to acknowledge the contributions of the many individuals and organizations that have provided support and encouragement for the project: Beverly J. McElmurry, EdD, FAAN, program director; Leo G. Niederman, MD, medical director; Gerusa Mello-Anderson, DDS, Ricardo Mendoza, DDS, and Indru Punwani, DDS, UIC College of Dentistry; Norman Katz, PhD, UIC College of Pharmacy; Lascelles Anderson, PhD, and Larry Nucci, PhD, principal investigators for the Nation of Tomorrow Project that was based in the UIC College of Education. Chicago Public Schools principals Karen Kerr, Lawrence McDougald, Donald Prather, Jacqueline Robinson, and Sylvia Rodriguez, along with assistant principals Paul Butler and Luz Gonzalez, have been welcoming and visionary in their work with the project.

Most important, the daily efforts of the project nurses, pediatricians, and school-community advocates must be recognized as the key ingredients of successful school health programs. Their competence, care, and concern have served as a model of what comprehensive school health programs can contribute to the learning environment of Chicago's elementary schools. Most recent team members working in the schools are Nurses Tekla Labovsky and Zoila Ortega; School-Community Advocates Luisita Collazo, Tasha Coursey, Nayda Hernandez, and Vivian Price; and Pediatricians Patricia Tibbs and Virginia Bishop-Townsend.

Earlier team members who contributed much to the development of the programs are Nurses Concepcion Favela, Marjorie Gadson, Ada Gonzalez, Glenda Huff, Georgann Karantonis, Colleen Lawlor, Helen Moore, and Johnetta Sisto; School-Community Advocates Sandra Alvarez, Judith Carabez, Theora Humphrey, Ursula Hunt, Sandra Inostroza, Mildred Martinez, Janice Overstreet, Rosa Ramirez, and Lisa Williams; and Pediatricians Susan Aquila, Mabel Blackwell, Charlene Gaebler, and Joyce Smith.

Last, but far from least, we must acknowledge the extraordinary technical skills, patience, and moral support provided by project secretaries Elsa Almaguer, Betty Jasper, and Donna Ruhl. They have done much to help us deal with the accounting and personnel systems of two highly complex organizational structures. Project research assistants Sharif Islam, Mary Maryland, and Simin Shekarloo also contributed a mix of talents: computer skills, critical inquiry, and most of all, enthusiasm.

INTRODUCTION

Increasing concern about the health and social problems that keep children from realizing their full potential has prompted many human service workers to consider schools as appropriate sites for providing a variety of support services. In Chicago, several inner-city elementary schools have developed school health centers that serve as the home base for orchestrating comprehensive school health programs designed to improve the chances for success of their students.

This chapter describes the relative merits of developing such school health programs based on the concepts of primary health care (PHC), that is, the extent to which the programs increase access to essential services; foster community participation in the schools' health programs; promote parent, student, and staff self-reliance; and develop intersectoral collaboration among health, social service, and governmental agencies responsible for the children's well-being.

The basic strategy employed in this project was to base multidisciplinary teams in two public elementary schools to address the health concerns that are a priority in each community. The teams consist of a full-time nurse, two school-community advocates, and a pediatrician who comes to the school one-half day per week. They are assisted with their health programs by faculty, fellows, and students from the colleges of dentistry, pharmacy, nursing, and social work.

The role of the school-community advocate is of particular importance in linking the team, especially the healthcare professionals, with the school, the parents, and with community resources. Because they are recruited from the immediate vicinity of the school, the advocates are very familiar with the culture of the school, the neighborhood, and share the general values and priorities of their neighbors.

The PHC teams complement the part-time service that is currently available in the schools to carry out the activities that are mandated by laws of the State of Illinois. Specifically, children must receive a complete and timely battery of immunizations; periodic screening for hearing and vision problems; physical examinations before moving into kindergarten, fifth, and ninth grades; and children with special health needs must receive timely assessment and planning for an educational program that is appropriate for their problems.

While this might seem to be a generous healthcare package by some standards, it falls short of meeting the actual needs of Chicago's children. The Chicago Public Schools (CPS) system serves over 400,000 students and employs approximately 225 nurses. Few schools have a full-time social worker and truant officers have been eliminated because of budget constraints. In addition to the health problems of children, Chicago is a port of entry for immigrants from many countries and their adjustment to a new way of life (e.g., climate, food, language, employment) affects children and their adjustment in school.

HEALTH OF CHILDREN

In many ways, the health of the nation's children has been improving steadily since the beginning of the twentieth century. Advances in medical technology, sanitation, availability of food and shelter, and general health knowledge of the citizenry have meant that middle- and upper-income families enjoy longer and healthier lives than their parents' generation. But for many families living in poverty in the inner cities and rural counties of the United States, progress is uneven or nonexistent.

In a recent assessment summarizing national progress in meeting the goals set for Healthy People 2000, researchers reported that 19 percent of the health indicators were proceeding in the wrong direction and that 3 percent remained unchanged. Unfortunately, "The proportion proceeding in the wrong direction is considerably greater for minorities" (McGinnis & Lee, 1995, p.1125). For blacks, asthma hospitalizations, adolescent pregnancies, AIDS incidence, and homicides continue to rise. Among Hispanics, AIDS, tuberculosis, homicides, and the prevalence of overweight women are also retreating from the Year 2000 targets.

The health status of children in Illinois and Chicago reflect these health trends as well as the so called new morbidities (e.g., emotional problems, abuse and neglect, drug abuse). As Table 1 indicates, one-third of Chicago's children live in poverty, which is nearly double the rate for Illinois (16.8 percent) and for the nation (17.9 percent). A disproportionate number of Chicago's children are also born into families at risk, a term defined by Voices for Illinois Children as having a teenage mother who is unmarried and without a high school diploma.

> Such families, because of emotional or economic instability, may be susceptible to hardships that heighten risks of child abuse and neglect, family disintegration, and children living with unmet special needs.
> . . . In isolation, any one of these factors may not destabilize a new family. But together these three risk factors...can be overwhelming. (Voices for Illinois Children, 1994, p. 12)

Concern about these and other problems affecting children and families has prompted health and social service professionals to consider schools as

TABLE 1.
Quality of Life Indicators in Chicago, Illinois, and the United States

Indicator	Chicago	Illinois	USA
Median family income	$30,707	$38,664	$32,772
Unemployment	9.2%	7.5%	7.4%
Children in poverty	33.3%	16.8%	17.9%
Infant mortality rate	13.3%	10.0%	8.4%
New families at risk	20.3%	12.6%	11.0%

Source: Voices for Illinois Children, 1994

appropriate sites from which to administer services designed to ameliorate many of the health and social problems that keep children from realizing their full potential (Adler & Gardner, 1994; Dryfoos, 1994; Igoe & Giordano, 1992). The University of Illinois at Chicago (UIC) is engaged in efforts to demonstrate how a land grant university can use its resources to strengthen and improve the institutions that directly serve children in urban areas through a cluster of special projects called the Nation of Tomorrow. Since 1989, with combined support from UIC, the W. K. Kellogg Foundation, and the Robert Wood Johnson Foundation, faculty and staff have worked with community agencies and residents on behalf of children. They developed plans and shared responsibilities for conducting programs aimed at assisting families, schools, and youth-serving agencies to

- increase pro-social behavior
- improve academic achievement
- increase awareness and adoption of healthy behavior
- decrease self-destructive behavior and increase children's sense of self-worth

HEALTH PROGRAM COMPONENTS

The work of the primary health care teams that are connected to these goals falls into three general categories: providing health services, providing health education, and engaging in community networking to build relationships with parents and local providers to involve them in the school's health program. The proportion of effort devoted to these general categories varies and depends on the unique characteristics of each school. For instance, one of the schools in the UIC project serves slightly over 1,400 students from a multicultural (83% Latino, 12% black, 1% Asian, and 3% white) and multi-socioeconomic status (SES) catchment area. The health center tallies approximately forty encounters per day, most of which are minor complaints but some of which warrant careful assessment, counseling, referral, and follow-up.

The other school, which serves 680 students, nearly all of whom are African American, has fewer daily encounters but maintains a heavier schedule of counseling, classroom presentations, teacher inservices, and parent sessions. The team also provides much more service to the school staff, largely in the form of screening and monitoring. Table 2 outlines examples of program activities and illustrates possibilities for engaging community residents as well as the staff of local health and/or service agencies in the school's health program.

ACCESS TO ESSENTIAL SERVICES

A priority voiced by each school's administration has been to have all students in compliance with state mandates for immunizations and school physical examinations. Full compliance ensures that no students will be excluded from school at the mid-October deadline and that their programs of study will not be interrupted because of this rule. This is especially important for students

TABLE 2.
Examples of School-based PHC Program Components

Health Services	Health Education	Community Networking
Students	*Classroom Topics*	Visit agencies.
First aid	Hand washing	Compile directory of
Immunization	First aid	local services and
School physical	Dental hygiene	resources.
examinations	Personal hygiene and	Update directory
Sports physical	grooming	annually.
examinations	Safety: fire, traffic,	Participate in health
Health fairs	home alone	coalitions.
Home visiting	Nutrition	Assist with local health
Counseling		fairs.
Referral and	*Parent Sessions*	Serve on advisory
follow-up	AIDS/STDs	boards.
Medication	Asthma	
administration	CPR	
Case management	Nutrition	
	Arthritis	
	Attention deficit	
	disorders	
Staff	*Teacher In-Services*	
Screenings:	Universal precautions	
blood pressure	for blood-borne	
glucose	pathogens	
cholesterol	Hepatitis	
Mantoux tests	Attention deficit	
	disorders	
	Seizure disorders	
	Stress management	
	Asthma	
	Diabetes	
	Nutrition	

entering ninth grade because absenteeism for any reason can sometimes be the first step in dropping out of school altogether. To address this, some principals require that students meet state-mandated requirements for physical examinations and immunizations before receiving their eighth grade diplomas.

Another important service is the follow-up of identified health problems. Common problems range from failing hearing, vision, or dental screenings to asthma, sickle cell anemia, seizure disorders, pregnancy, suspected abuse or neglect, or mental health problems. While screenings, immunizations, and selected primary care problems can be managed by the pediatricians during their weekly consultations, other problems are referred to local providers or to the appropriate university clinic. The teams subscribe to the notion of promoting continuity of care in a "medical home" whenever this is possible. By this we mean obtaining services from a provider who maintains a child's full health history and who can manage care that is beyond the scope of the health center's capabilities.

But even when referrals are made and students receive care at local facilities, they sometimes return to the health center for supplementary advice. For instance, an eigth grader with a confirmed diagnosis of an STD sought answers to numerous questions: How did he get it? Could he have passed it to his girlfriend or did he get it from her? Did she need treatment? What type of protection should they use? And, who was to blame?

HEALTH EDUCATION

In addition to classroom sessions for the students, team members respond to requests from teachers, parents, the school administration, and the community to provide information about health-related topics of special concern to them. For instance, teachers at a nearby school requested help with stress management when their school was placed on a list of schools needing remediation because of students' low test scores. At another school, the team's nurse and physician conducted a series of nine classes for neighborhood parents on a variety of health topics.

Both schools provide screening and monitoring services for parents and staff, some of whom have chronic conditions that are distressing to them. In one instance, a mother was caring for her husband who had suffered a stroke. Because she too had high blood pressure, she was concerned that she might have a stroke. The regular monitoring she receives at the health center reassures her that her medication is effective.

The school-community advocates also participate in each team's health education programs by providing classroom presentations. Popular topics include handwashing, dental hygiene, safety and first aid, basic nutrition, and personal hygiene and grooming. They also spearheaded community-oriented programs on the proper use of automobile safety seats as well as advocacy for parents with immigration or housing problems, or who need public assistance.

The advocates report that the experience of preparing and presenting these lessons contributes not only to their personal knowledge, but also sometimes uncovers latent talents and strengths. Indeed, several of them have moved on to institutions of higher education or to positions in community agencies.

COMMUNITY NETWORKING

As we noted earlier, an important function of each school's health center team is to ensure that there is follow-up of identified health problems. In order to accomplish this, staff have conducted their own community assessments to become acquainted with local providers and services. They have compiled directories listing a broad range of agencies, associations, churches, and programs that might be of use to families of students. The directories are updated annually during the summer and copies are shared with local agencies as well as other members of the school staff.

While the compilation and distribution of the directories serve a useful purpose in facilitating referrals, the process of information gathering also fosters the development of linkages and cooperation within the community. The most visible example of this effort occurs when the teams organize health fairs or community resource fairs for students and parents. A number of agency representatives volunteer their services for screenings such as blood pressure, cholesterol, and diabetes, and provide informational material about their services. Also, during the fair they visit among themselves and with school staff and parents, thus contributing to network development, a distinguishing feature of PHC.

A closely related principle that some analysts consider to be the cornerstone of PHC (Rifkin, 1996; Sawyer, 1995; White & Wehlage, 1995) is community participation. In our experience, it has been the most challenging principle to put into practice. The teams have attempted to recruit advisory boards, based on the belief that developing such boards will ensure that each school's program is tailored to the unique needs and concerns of its own community. Ideally, board members invest time, ideas, resources, and personal commitment in building a sustainable health center that is responsive to the school community. In principle, this investment on the part of community residents should result in a sense of ownership of the center and its programs, and a willingness to advocate for incorporating it into the infrastructure of the school system and the community.

CONCLUSION

Even though the programs that we have described thus far are operational in only a handful of Chicago public schools, the process of developing and launching them has taught us some lessons about the complexity of such an undertaking. If this effort is to be mounted on a larger scale, and particularly if the programs incorporate the principles of PHC, these lessons warrant consideration.

The prospect of facilitating access to health services is paramount when school administrators and parents consider locating a health center in their school. For most students, parents, teachers, and school staff, school-based health centers are ideal for connecting students, and sometimes parents, with the services they need and want. They value the availability of on-site vaccinations and physical examinations, services that expedite enrollment of students and the recruitment of parent volunteers. Immigrant families and those burdened with social problems benefit especially when they are spared waiting for an appointment and/or a trip to a clinic.

In one instance, a mother with a positive reaction to her tuberculin test was helped to get an immediate appointment for further evaluation. A school-community advocate accompanied her to assist with language barriers. In the course of the trip, the mother confided that her husband did not like her to leave the house and that at times he was abusive. The team was able to share information about her rights as well as possible sources of protection.

Convenience aside, however, team members must be sensitive to the importance of encouraging families to develop continuing relationships with a medical home. Acting as a broker to form linkages with local providers fosters the intersectoral collaboration that must be addressed as health centers are planned. There is a natural tendency, especially among agencies, to compete for resources, turf, and recognition. This competitive milieu often displaces even the most altruistic objectives, particularly when the outcomes and rewards are uncertain. Participants must be willing to expend a great deal of time and good will in building trust and maintaining dialogue with a variety of agencies and disciplines if school-based health centers are to become an integral part of the community's healthcare system without becoming a burden for an already stressed school system.

A related lesson concerns identifying grassroots individuals to participate in the planning and implementation of the health centers. Unfortunately, there does not seem to be a tradition of social activism on issues of child health in most inner-city communities. Rather, parents and other residents experience competing priorities for their time and resources by issues such as employment, housing, and safety. As a consequence, team members must make special efforts to identify and engage neighbors who can voice grass-roots community sentiment and perspectives on what they want their school health program to be. Active participation in the process provides a unique opportunity for learning about how the healthcare and school systems work. This in turn has the potential for broader community development efforts as community residents develop knowledge, skills, and confidence in dealing with administrative officials.

Finally an obstacle to introducing PHC programs is the lack of resources for community-based services. This is, in part, the result of resource allocation within the U.S. healthcare system that favors sophisticated technology oriented toward curing disease versus preventing it. A related obstacle is the scarcity of data that would clarify the relative benefits of a broader spectrum of prevention measures. For example, a great deal of attention is given to the cost savings of childhood immunization and oral rehydration for infant diarrhea. But equally important is the need to evaluate the long-term benefits of many other measures that could be orchestrated in schools, such as comprehensive health education, dental care, and life-long exercise.

In this regard, program staff are paying closer attention to documenting their activities and keeping records of services provided. This is beneficial as a marketing tool for school health programs and as a database for research about the effects of the program on students and staff. As a means of increasing access to services, several small-scale studies have been undertaken by faculty and students of the health professions in the areas of homelessness, violence prevention, community empowerment, and health fairs.

We anticipate that as the programs mature and become stabilized within their individual schools, they will become steady practicum sites for students from all of the health professions. Currently a dental fellow-in-training is providing a dental sealant program for second and sixth graders at one school while at another school a pediatric fellow is studying the health needs of children in unstable housing situations as well as providing primary care services. In addition, nursing students at the graduate and undergraduate levels are participating in screening, counseling, and health education activities at both schools.

We should point out, however, that the task of reorienting faculty from their traditional views about preparing health profession students for providing acute care in hospital settings is an uphill battle. Unfortunately, it is reinforced by concerns of parents when they learn that their college students are based in community sites in the inner city. On the other hand, schools welcome the contributions that students of the health professions (as well as student teachers) make to their schools.

Clearly, inner-city schools provide fertile ground for launching PHC initiatives. Not only do schools provide a focal point for community activity and serve as a forum for discussion of community concerns, they are a readily accessible site for delivering a variety of services tailored to the unique needs and desires of urban communities. It is our hope that the reform efforts that seek to restructure both the healthcare and the education systems will recognize the value of incorporating health and social service support systems into local community schools.

The words of Irving Harris (1992), an ardent spokesman for Chicago's children, remind us of the importance of persevering in efforts to operationalize PHC in urban settings:

> Children are the future of the world. We owe it to them to ensure that they are born with the best possible chance to live, love, grow, and excel. If we shirk this responsibility we will have contributed directly to the misery and suffering of generations to come. If we fulfil this obligation, we will have given the world a gift of inestimable value. (p. 24)

REFERENCES

Adler, L. & Gardner, S. (Eds.). (1994). The politics of linking schools and social services: The 1993 yearbook of the Politics of Education Association. Washington, D.C.: Falmer Press.

Dryfoos, J. (1994). Full-service schools: A revolution in health and social services for children, youth, and families. San Francisco: Jossey-Bass.

Harris, I. B. (1992). Primary prevention vs. intervention. In *Focus on children: The beat of the future*. Conference conducted at the Columbia University Graduate School of Journalism. New York, N. Y.

Igoe, J. B. & Giordano, B. P. (1992). *Expanding school health services to serve families in the 21st century*. Washington, D. C.: American Nurses Publishing.

McGinnis, J. M. & Lee, P. R. (1995). Healthy People 2000 at mid-decade. *JAMA, 273*(14), 1123–1129.

Redlener, D. (1997, April). *Access: What is it and what needs to be done?* Paper presented at the National Interdisciplinary Conference on Access to Primary Health Care, Chicago, IL.

Rifkin, S. B. (1996). Paradigms lost: Toward a new understanding of community participation in health programmes. *Acta Tropica, 61,* 79–92.

Sawyer, L. M. (1995). Community participation: Lip service? *Nursing Outlook, 43,* 17–22.

Voices for Illinois Children. (1994). Chicago kids count: Community by community profiles of child well-being. Chicago: Author.

White, J. A. & Wehlage, G. (1995). Community collaboration: If it is such a good idea, why is it so hard to do? *Education Evaluation and Policy Analysis, 17*(1), 23–38.

Chapter 16

Primary Health Care Curriculum for Urban School Children: Grades K–8

BEVERLY J. MCELMURRY
B. JOAN NEWCOMB
AGATHA LOWE
SUSAN J. MISNER

Project Dates: January 1992–March 1996
The project was partially funded by Otho S. A. Sprague Memorial Foundation and the UIC College of Nursing.

This chapter describes a primary health care (PHC) curriculum for grades K–8 that was developed and introduced in selected Chicago public schools. Using a PHC approach, we engaged community residents, school personnel, students, and their parents in identifying their health concerns and interests, and in turn incorporated these concerns into the health education curriculum. The assumption was that a health curriculum is more likely to increase health knowledge and reduce health risk behaviors if it includes health topic issues that are important to the learners.

OBJECTIVES

The specific objectives of the project were as follows:

1. Involve the school community in the identification of health concerns.
2. Design a health curriculum that students could use to promote and maintain their health and/or manage illness and chronic conditions.
3. Implement and evaluate an age- and needs-appropriate PHC curriculum for school-age children (grades K–8) and their families.
4. Collaborate with community-based organizations in the development of community structures to maintain a PHC curriculum network for inner-city school children.
5. Disseminate information about the curriculum to Chicago schools' personnel and communities.

BACKGROUND

The curriculum project was developed as a supplement to a K–8 school-based health services program described in the previous chapter. In the process of introducing school-based services we emphasized that PHC is an approach to health care that focuses on the promotion of health and the prevention of diseases through comprehensive care that is collaborative and cooperatively provided by community people and multiple professional disciplines. PHC is interactive. Community residents are encouraged to be knowledgeable in health matters and to have an opportunity to participate in their healthcare management. Moreover, PHC addresses self-care practices for physical and mental aspects of community health as well as community, social, and environmental conditions. A basic goal is to ensure that PHC is available to everyone in the community.

The Chicago School Reform Movement that started in the late 1980s encouraged school innovation, and it was within this climate that the PHC curriculum developed. The policy of the Chicago Board of Education was to support the autonomous development of programs that met the specific needs of the students in a particular school or community. Principals, teachers, and parents (through the Local School Council) and community organizations were encouraged to identify and address the health and academic needs of the students.

CHICAGO CLUSTER INITIATIVE

The first three years (1992–1995) of the curriculum development project were funded by the Otho S. A. Sprague Foundation via a grant to the Chicago Cluster Initiative. The University of Illinois at Chicago (UIC) College of Nursing, Partners in Health (PIH) program was subcontracted to develop the curriculum. The Cluster Initiative was composed of representatives from the city's housing, parks, and schools areas. These representative groups were drawn from public and not-for-profit agencies in the city of Chicago. Their joint goal was to create a first-rate educational experience for 24,000 children and their families in four community areas, or clusters, in Chicago, using both public and private resources within and outside the public schools. The cluster intent was to realign and redistribute the combined resources of cluster partners in order to improve educational outcomes, guaranteeing those school children entry in solid post-secondary education or jobs. Each cluster area was defined as a high school and its feeder elementary schools. Table 1 presents data on one cluster area that was selected for initial curriculum development. Chicago politics are never static and the subsequent changes in leadership in the component areas (i.e., park, school, and housing) resulted in frequent changes in the staff and focus of the Cluster Initiative. By the third year of the project, the university-based personnel were the only component working on curriculum development.

Chicago Public Schools. The implementation of health education programs in the public schools in the city of Chicago reflects the national norm. The comprehensive curriculum guide had not been revised for several years, and most schools did not use it. Instead, separate curricula for Family Life Education, Drug Education, and AIDS Education had been substituted in its place. In addition, a variety of agencies or educational institutions were often invited to present health classes in the schools. The more popular of these being nutrition, dental health, and fire and accident prevention. The curricula from the Board of Education were recommended rather than mandated, and decisions to implement curricula were at the discretion of the principal, teachers, and local school council. (In Chicago, a local school council is the equivalent of a school board for each school).

The project staff took the position that an integral part of improving educational outcomes is to equip students with tools that allow them to make decisions about their health even when they are suffering from chronic illness. Even though the children were receiving health information prior to our collaborative endeavor, there was concern about the lack of continuity from year to year in the health topics presented to the students and the lack of health knowledge and skills students were acquiring. The limited school finances and number of health professionals available to teach school-based health courses resulted in the decision that regular classroom teachers should be equipped with tools that would make them the major health educators of the students.

TABLE 1.
Demographics for One Chicago School Cluster
Selected for Initial Curriculum Development

Curriculum Demonstration Community[*]			
Total population	114,079	Population aged 0–24	44%
Racial/ethnic composition: **Black Latino White** 86% 4% 9%		Population under 18 living in poverty (compared to a U.S. average of 21%)	35%
Population in poverty (compared to a U.S. average of 14%)	26%	Teenage births	25%
Population on some form of public aid	38%	Students low-income (1991–1992) (compared to a state average of 32%)	64%
Population unemployed	18%	Graduation Rate (1991–1992) (compared to a state average of 81%)	18%
Unoccupied housing	11%	High school attendance rate (1991–1992) (compared to a state average of 94%)	69%

[*] These statistics were compiled from the City of Chicago Department of Planning and Development—Policy, Research and Planning Division, the Chicago Department of Public Health—Division of Health Systems and Statistics, and school report card data. Data are for 1990 and represent the Chicago Austin community that was selected for project focus. The Chicago Cluster Initiative selected school communities for their high concentration of low-income children, low graduation rates and geographic diversity.

A doctorally prepared nurse with expertise in health education and PHC and a community health liaison worker employed to develop the curriculum met with personnel at a school serving African-American students. Through focus groups with teachers and parents, this nurse/advocate team elicited health-related concerns of urban, multiethnic children. This information was used to identify and develop health content for the curriculum.

THE PRIMARY HEALTH CARE (PHC) CURRICULUM

The resulting health education curriculum (the primary health care curriculum for urban school children) used a comprehensive health education approach. The curriculum consists of 36–42 weekly lesson plans for each grade that cover topics in the following ten categories:

- Prevention and control of diseases
- Growth and development
- Drug abuse prevention
- Safety and first aid
- Consumer awareness
- Family health
- Human sexuality
- Community health
- Mental health
- Nutrition

The curriculum includes items of information for parents so that they can reinforce what their children are learning in the school. In addition, the curriculum is designed to be integrated into each teacher's overall curriculum plan on a weekly basis. The ten themes are elaborated upon each year so that the depth of student knowledge builds as they progress from grade to grade. The desired outcomes of the curriculum were to prepare students with the following:

- Knowledge, skills, and attitudes that promote health-enhancing activities benefitting them, their families, and their community
- An understanding of their responsibilities as students and as community residents to contribute to the health of their environment
- Information that helps them to examine a variety of career options in the health field
- The initial self-confidence, interpersonal skills, and awareness they will need to function well in a family context, as well as in a changing society

As we introduced the curriculum into a sample of schools in the CPS system we learned that there is a need for teacher preparation to effectively implement the curriculum. While some teachers were unfamiliar or uncomfortable with certain health topics, others did not see the value of incorporating basic health information and practice in classroom activities.

The curriculum for health education and promotion combined with school-based/linked health services represented a comprehensive health program. In essence, a comprehensive program uses community-based PHC and social service approaches. Academic and service professionals work as partners with community residents to address child health and welfare issues. The locus of these efforts in the local public school represents the selection of a site that people can access and adapt when they collaborate to design and carry out programs that will help students achieve academically and develop physically and socially.

ACCOMPLISHMENTS

While the implementation and evaluation of a K–8 PHC curriculum for inner-city children continues to be a focus of our activity, the following were accomplished during a $3\frac{1}{2}$-year period:

- Conducted and evaluated results of focus groups with parents, principals, teachers, and students of primarily African-American school communities in two K–8 elementary schools and a high school to determine health needs and interests of stakeholders in those settings
- Assessed the health-related concerns and interests of teachers and school resource personnel through survey distribution and analysis in five K–8 urban elementary schools
- Developed a core comprehensive health curriculum tailored to the identified health needs/interests of urban school children, grades K–8[1]
- Tested a participatory design for evaluation of teachers' satisfaction with the curriculum in one elementary school
- Modified and adapted the K–8 curriculum after conducting a pilot implementation in one school (K–8)
- Disseminated the PHC curriculum to elementary schools in Chicago for review by the administrative/teaching staff and/or parent groups and mailed the curriculum or segments of it to those who requested copies. Some agencies used the curriculum without our awareness when they heard about it from others in the community
- Familiarized parents and teachers in selected schools with available health education resources and involved them in the critique and selection of health education materials/resources
- Involved university students and programs as participants in providing school-based health education. This included nursing students, family practice residents, Chicago Health Corps (an AmeriCorps Program) participants, and undergraduate honors program students
- Collaborated with community-based organizations to promote community support for comprehensive school health education

---

[1]The physical attributes of the curriculum are that it was prepared as a nine-volume set of specific grade lesson plans. Thus for each grade level (K–8) there is a separate notebook with roughly 36–42 lesson plans for each grade. Initially we reviewed the Michigan Model of Health Education to see if it could be used in Chicago, but the schools and project personnel judged it as only partially appropriate to our situation. Therefore, while we leaned heavily on the experience in Michigan, our K–8 curriculum combined the racial/ethnic concerns that emerged in focus groups and trial activities as well as out of concern that the curriculum incorporate PHC emphases.

- Identified a speaker's bureau or resource list of experts on health and educational topics to foster linkage relationships between local community service organizations, the PHC curriculum project, and partner-participating health education schools
- Conducted ongoing local community education and public relations activities such as a joint fundraising activity with five participating K–8 school partners at a Chicago restaurant, sponsored exhibition tables at school open houses, and community development meetings with a local hospital and approximately twenty different local agencies
- Collaborated with the National League for Nursing (New York) in production of a videotape on community programs for youth, *Children's Health in the Community.* This video is commercially available and illustrates national programs that work to improve children's health
- Participated and contributed to coalition development in the comprehensive school health education field on both local and national levels (see Table 1 in previous chapter for list of collaborative groups)

CONTINUING CONCERNS

The work thus far with students, parents, teachers, and other educators, has provided insights about comprehensive health education. Although we have focused on a local level, the global perspective on school health is consistent with our experience. The World Health Organization (WHO), through an Expert Committee on Comprehensive School Health Education and Promotion, has identified a Global School Health Initiative to:

1. Document expert recommendations on policy and action steps which can be taken to improve health through schools and communities
2. Convince policy-makers of the benefits of investing in health programs in schools
3. Gather evidence of effective ways to improve the health of school-aged children, their families, and school staffs through schools
4. Develop major strategies to implement and institutionalize school health programs

Over the course of the PHC curriculum project, the faculty/staff and school administrators/teachers from partner schools have expanded their insight regarding the driving forces and constraints in achieving "health" as an integral component of children's education. To meet the learning needs of urban school children, core content in a comprehensive health education curriculum must be broad based. Health knowledge and health skills are built upon a wide range of critical substantive themes over the course of time, both within a child's grade year, and across different grade levels. The resultant incremental "education" is designed to positively influence the health choices/ decisions and health behavior of individual students, as well as their overall academic achievement and life course.

While the effectiveness of comprehensive health education for school children might be considered intuitively beneficial, there is inadequate documentation of benefits by research. Given the incremental nature of a comprehensive approach to health education, we appreciate the challenge posed by efforts to measure the benefits of health curricula for children that capture health-related outcomes overtime. Thus, until comprehensive data are available, any benefit attributable from health education for an aggregate of children may be perceived by educators as intangible and transitory.

A presumptive view by educators of health lessons as "fluff" content is intensified when the public mandate emphasizes accountability for basic literacy and mathematics competencies. This is particularly true in school systems where this standard of quality education has not been achieved and the jobs of teachers and administrators are threatened if students do not achieve desired levels on standard tests. In response to educators' accountability for students' attainment of basic reading and mathematics skills, the relationship may be obscured between the health knowledge, health skills, and health status of students and those students' achievement of traditional educational goals.

LESSONS LEARNED

Given the above, the following material offers a summary of constraints encountered during the development, implementation, and evaluation of the PHC curriculum to date, as well as approaches we have taken to counter these barriers:

- **There is a perception within the educational community that the public mandate for assurance of a student's literacy and mathematics skills dictates a narrowing of educational system focus and restricts the role of school personnel regarding the health and social services needs of students and their families.** We maintain that health personnel have a role in public education regarding the relationship between children's academic achievement and their self-care/healthcare resources, health knowledge, and health skills. Thus, health professionals must assist schools to broaden their service capacity through linkage with an increasing array of service programs/providers and university/college partners. Comprehensive school health education programs are strengthened when there is a parallel and strong comprehensive school health services program. It is important that PHC curriculum staff conduct public relations efforts to emphasize that "being healthy helps kids learn." Through the participation of volunteer groups such as the Chicago Health Corps, it is possible to identify local community service programs and health providers accessible to the PHC partner school's children and their families. Collaborative school partners assure cohesiveness of the PHC curriculum and the school's overall health program.
- **The primary education system has limited appreciation for "health science" as a legitimate academic area of study for elementary students, or for promoting opportunities to integrate basic science and social science content within a health science curriculum.** As a distinct

and growing body of knowledge, health science is applicable and pertinent to the education of America's school children. The inclusion of health science as an integral content area for primary education is important and can be achieved through the integration of relevant "health" content into class sessions on related basic and social science course content. It is important that PHC curriculum faculty and staff consult on an ongoing basis with administrators and teachers at the project's partner schools to identify the process for curriculum inclusion in a specific school setting. Those teachers who have most successfully used the PHC curriculum have identified methods to integrate the "health lessons" into their weekly lesson plans. Where class content is "compartmentalized" or "departmentalized," as is often common in the upper-division grades (seventh and eighth), the inclusion of a health curriculum has been more arduous. The level of health information required for mastery by both teachers and students is likely to be a factor that constrains implementation of the health curriculum in upper-division grades.

■ **Indigenous hazards and crime in the immediate environs of many schools elicit a protectionist response from some local school councils and administrators that risk isolating schools as "islands within their own communities," increasingly disengaged from beneficial community resources.** While supporting security measures that protect school children from crime and hazards, health personnel can also assist school administrators, teachers, and parents to collaborate with concerned community residents in community-wide violence prevention initiatives. Our PHC curriculum staff surveys of teachers clearly demonstrated their concern about the students' safety from crime, especially gangs and violence. Through school inservice programs/meetings, PHC curriculum staff use opportunities to introduce school administrators/staff to other community programs to address community violence. Also, through orientation to the lesson modules of the PHC curriculum, such as conflict resolution, self-esteem, and "emotional intelligence," teachers are provided resources to assist students in learning alternatives to violence in solving conflicts and problems.

■ **The experience and preparation of elementary school classroom teachers for implementing health education curriculum is disparate.** The PHC curriculum personnel surveyed the teaching staff at some partner schools regarding the interests/needs of teachers for health information. Based on an analysis of these surveys, inservice training sessions were offered to address the teachers' priority concerns about "health education." Qualified presenters from the university and from local community-based organizations also conducted training sessions. There is a need to expand the quality and extent of health sciences education in the university/college programs that prepare teachers for elementary and secondary schools. Multidisciplinary partnerships between university health sciences, teacher preparation, and curriculum development programs are one means we would like to see tried in future preparation of K–8 teachers.

- **There are limits in the health professional's awareness of the structure and organizational culture of the elementary and secondary educational system.** Turmoil and upheaval in the organization and structure of a public school system attracts attention from local media, and often garners unfavorable public attention. The development of "partnerships" in a rapidly changing environment requires formation of collegial trust between external school personnel and partner school/community staff. The formation of these institutional and personnel relationships must frequently overcome a view of university academic/personnel as, at best, "invited guests" and, at worst, "intrusive outsiders" to the school setting and in some cases to the community. One principal's question, "What do you bring to the party?" illustrates the skepticism of some school administrators about the potential contribution of university personnel to school initiatives. In our experience, the PHC curriculum implementation required an investment of time, energy, and persistence in negotiating meeting schedules, clarifying project goals and objectives, and reconciling the goals of the curriculum with other school-based initiatives. Due to the uniqueness of each school's administrative division of responsibilities, organizational differentiation, and particular human and material resources, a lengthy and rigorous process of developing a specific strategic plan with each partner school is necessary prior to implementation of the curriculum.

- **The decision to use a "comprehensive school health curriculum" can be perceived as a rejection of "focused health curricula."** Educational systems continually redefine their role and priorities in addressing the educational needs of school children. The assessment of potential benefit to students from specific programs and curricula represent a response to an array of criteria, including political pressure, parent demands, and immediate situational crises. From a viewpoint of limited resources (i.e., human, material, and time), a health curriculum that is comprehensive and broad based risks being viewed by school personnel as duplicative of previously selected "focused topic" curricula, such as substance abuse or conflict resolution. Focused curricula on specific health-related issues of particular concern to teachers and school administrators can be included but does not substitute for the development of fundamental health knowledge and health skills that are necessary for informed and sound health decision making and behavior over the course of a child's school years and into adulthood. During the course of the PHC curriculum project, there were continued efforts by the project personnel to clarify the desired outcomes of a comprehensive approach to the health education of school children. This process resulted in project personnel and school staff identification of new applications/adaptations of the PHC curriculum for specific target groups, such as preschoolers, children in special education classes, and extended day programs.

CONCLUSION

The ultimate effect of the above changes on the curriculum project was that our original partner, the Cluster Initiative (i.e., parks, housing, and schools components) was dissolved and lost to the project. In large urban settings, each public school is considered part of a larger school bureaucracy, but in reality most of them survive as fairly self-contained, isolated, and underfunded units. Most change and innovation seem to proceed school by school according to the energy and skill of local personnel.

The importance of invigorating health education in urban schools remains a concern and an area for national attention. Further, it is important to focus evaluation on both the processes and outcomes entailed in introducing a comprehensive health curriculum to teachers, promoting its use, and determining its effectiveness in enhancing students' health knowledge and behaviors.

In our experience, frequent changes in the leadership of major city government service areas has been an aspect of the urban experience that makes continuity of projects difficult and unpredictable. For us, it is important that our partnerships reflect the levels of an urban academic health center that seek to provide technical resources and assistance to the communities that it serves in a respectful and collaborative fashion. It is in the best interests of everyone to ensure that urban children receive an education that maximizes their potential for healthy and productive lives. Perseverance is important and necessary to achieve desired goals.

REFERENCES

Moss, L. (1995). Video Producer. *Children's health in the community.* New York: NLN. (42-2712).

World Health Organization Fact Sheet. (1995). Comprehensive School Health Education and Promotion. *Fact Sheet, No. 92,* September. Geneva, Switzerland: WHO.

Chapter 17

Health Care and Community Health in the Current Environment

LINDA DIAMOND SHAPIRO
BENN GREENSPAN

As health care in Chicago has changed dramatically during the past few years, centers of healthcare giving—from doctors' offices to large institutions—have faced new financial pressures and management directives. The ownership of several healthcare entities has changed, sometimes several times within a short period. Many health institutions have altered or abandoned their original missions. Some have lost the essential connection that once existed with the communities they serve.

In this current environment, regardless of whether the purpose of healthcare delivery is defined as service or profit, all institutions retain the need to maintain their essential connection to local communities and local neighborhoods. Community health is a key managed care goal: If enough local patients are enrolled in a plan and served by a system of providers, the health of that community determines the financial fortunes of the plan.

This chapter explores possible economic relationships between healthcare institutions and the communities they serve. While providers and insurers have developed a comprehensive scholarly, professional, and trade literature describing goals and methods for addressing community health, a much smaller literature has sought to understand what makes a community healthy as defined by the community itself. Even more challenging has been the effort to find working models for collaboration between health institutions that serve surrounding low-income communities, and which attempt to improve economic vitality as a proxy for health.

The community development roles that community leaders may envision for health facilities may indeed be very far from traditional healthcare agendas. While community leaders may be looking for economic development resources, health facilities frequently focus their energies on disease and disability and on creating access for underserved community residents to healthcare services. Nevertheless, several trends in the Chicago environment have been calling health facilities and the communities they serve to address community-building from some new perspectives.

This chapter summarizes some of the wisdom and experience generated by a Chicago town meeting convened by the Sinai Health System on these subjects. Sinai Health System is a community-oriented provider of comprehensive health care for several of Chicago's medically underserved and economically devastated communities. Drawing on ideas generated during this town meeting, this summary provides some parameters for defining the broad context in which health institutions might serve as a partner in community development, with an emphasis on partnerships to fortify economically endangered neighborhoods.

HEALTH ACCESS AND COMMUNITY HEALTH

The healthcare delivery system in Chicago, as in other urban areas across the country, is currently restructuring itself to face an uncertain future environment characterized by the implementation of a mandatory managed care program within the state's chronically underfunded Medicaid program (Joseph, 1995), a welfare reform program, "immigration reform," and a newly reorganized state human service delivery system. All of this is occurring in the context of continued changes in commercial insurance coverage for the working population. These changes, which in some ways may represent improvements in health and human service systems, also send the clear signal that less public and private money will be available to support healthcare service delivery. At the same time, the number of uninsured keeps growing. It is all a message that indicates that health access barriers require redoubled attention.

In Chicago, while some basic indicators of access to care, such as childhood immunization rates, have demonstrably improved during the decade, other public health problems have grown as evidenced by increases in substance abuse, HIV, asthma, tuberculosis, hypertension, and sexually transmitted diseases. In Chicago, as across the nation, these problems disproportionately affect patients in poor neighborhoods for whom a range of environmental hardships compete for attention with health problems, while barriers to the few affordable health resources continue to grow higher and more numerous.

Lack of financial access to care is compounded in Chicago by the geographic isolation of poor residents from sources of care. Maintaining the supply of primary care providers in underserved areas remains a serious problem, accounting for the large number of medically underserved areas in the Chicago metropolitan area with particularly severe gaps for the uninsured poor, working poor, and their dependents.

Further, as private employers continue to seek discounts on the managed care products they purchase, less money is available for healthcare institutions in Chicago to provide care to Medicaid and unsponsored patients through cross-subsidies from private insurance. The federally sponsored community health centers in Chicago currently expect increased demand for unsponsored care as a result of these private market changes.

These trends in Chicago are local expressions of national issues. Medicaid restructuring, market changes, reductions in availability and extent of employer-based insurance, and nonfinancial barriers to care encountered by the underserved are ubiquitous in urban centers. Economically disadvantaged neighborhoods typically have high rates of health problems; not surprisingly, a downward economic spiral is often related to poor community health status. First, because good health is an important prerequisite for attaining an education and participating in the labor force, many ill people are not insured. Second, paradoxically, the labor force is one of the key portals of entry into the mainstream healthcare delivery system, so many unemployed people are at risk for diminished care and as a result, poor health, and chronic disease. Employer-based health insurance continues to provide the most certain guarantee of health access.

REFRAMED PERSPECTIVES ON THE HEALTH SYSTEM

These comments point in directions that may require fundamental changes in the ways that both privately and publicly funded programs address poverty in the context of existing institutional imperatives. The healthcare delivery system represents one example.

The continuing concentration of poor health status within defined neighborhoods provides a powerful argument for reorganizing and targeting health resources and services by communities. However, our financial and institutional systems are set up to provide a conventional mix of medical and social services, billed and budgeted on the basis of individual episodes of service, and to substitute acute care for prevention. In fact, health resources in our nation are primarily developed to provide illness intervention for a few (whether these services are prepaid or reimbursed on a fee-for-service basis). Common wisdom shows that "what gets done is what gets rewarded." The irony is that at a time when we can identify the increased need for attention to "health," the preponderance of our health resources are in a system being squeezed tightly to remove what it defines as unnecessary, that is, nonessential, noncritical care.

It should be no surprise, then, that within the rich web of existing public and private healthcare enterprises, the often-expressed interest in addressing community health status only rarely gets translated into an integrated plan of action. The challenge is to (1) define the case for building a healthier community, (2) articulate how serious attention to community health fits into the larger health marketplace and economic development activity underway, and (3) establish policy and organizational ideas for implementing a health-producing agenda, one that most likely takes economic health as its point of departure.

Report cards are becoming increasingly important tools for assessment and accountability in the healthcare delivery field. As healthcare delivery systems come to be held accountable for cost-effective approaches to achieving outcomes, the maxim "what gets measured gets done" is increasingly applicable. The notion of a "report card" for assessing community health requires creative thinking beyond the traditional health indicators typically assessed by public-health agencies and even beyond the ground-breaking work done in the Hospital and Community Benefit Standards Program sponsored by the Robert Wood Johnson Foundation in the late 1980s. While traditional indicators remain important for assessing and monitoring community health, less-traditional approaches also must be considered.

Traditional health status indicators include mortality rates, rates of infectious and chronic disease, and morbidity rates such as missed school days and days of productive life lost. However, in the context of community health, this list of indicators could look much different—it could be composed of indicators that serve as proxies for health status and go to the core of community life. Indicators that describe community infrastructure and human or social capital may indeed reflect the goal of maintaining and improving health, while recognizing the role of "group-or-community" health in the health of individuals.

A 1995 Sinai Health System town meeting, convened specifically to promote the thinking of community members outside of the health sector, generated a short list of these alternative health indicators. In the same spirit, a small Chicago project has sought to identify some actual definitions of community health generated by Chicago residents (Hojvat-Gallin, in press). Some of these indicators might include: integrity of social networks; education levels; environmental quality indicators; effectiveness of transportation resources; unemployment rates; domestic violence, street crime, and homicide rates; availability of police, fire department, and ambulances to respond to emergencies; cab driver safety; quality of public parks and public spaces; number of vacant lots; ratio of grocery stores with fresh food to stores that sell liquor and cigarettes; quality of housing stock; high school drop-out rates; literacy levels; proportion of community children placed in foster care; proportion of incarcerated community members; and proportion of children who eat breakfast before coming to school.

One value of a community-health report card is that these measures can be watched within the community. Local residents can mark progress toward improvements in these categories. While these nontraditional health-status concepts beg further definition and require further construction so they can be measured, they have considerable appeal for addressing community health in broad terms.

WISDOM FROM BEYOND
THE HEALTH SECTOR

Recognizing the economic resource that health institutions might serve for community development purposes (Greenspan, 1992; Manilow, 1994), the Sinai Health System convened a full-day town meeting in 1995 to celebrate its first anniversary as an integrated system consisting of Mount Sinai Hospital Medical Center, Schwab Rehabilitation Center, Sinai Community Institute, and the Sinai Medical Group. The reflections of the diverse participants in the Chicago town meeting provided a good inventory of issues and approaches that Chicagoans believe could be deployed to improve the "health" of communities, broadly defined. This inventory is summarized here as a point of departure for developing models for the collaborative work of community building.

Participants in this full-day discussion included local business owners, block club members, community-based organization leaders, tenants' organization members, and participants in church-based economic development programs. From the public sector, representatives included aldermen, a county board member, a Chicago Housing Authority official, Chicago Public Schools representatives, and city public health staff. Other participants included several representatives of local health policy and advocacy groups, a benefits manager of a *Fortune 500* firm, leadership from the state medical society, and a group of faculty from a range of health-related disciplines.

The discussion was facilitated by a number of nationally recognized academic leaders in community health, including John McKnight of Northwestern University, Dr. Helen Rodriguez-Trias, a former president of the American Public Health Association now consulting nationwide, and Edward Lawlor and Richard Sewell, both of the University of Chicago.

Both McKnight (1993, 1994) and Rodriguez-Trias (1993) are among the few educators who have developed research-based tools for mobilizing local residents into community health planning. Both point to some of the same key principles. Definitions of the health of a community can only be achieved if everyone in the community is truly present or soundly represented. An understanding of the combined capacities of everyone in the community should serve as the starting point for planning. Traditional planning tools such as needs assessments are frequently irrelevant to community health, because they fail to identify resources that can fuel community health.

These principles set the tone for the observations of the conferees on the broad issues of jobs, education, economic development, access to healthcare, and housing. Recommendations and quotes from this day included the following:

Health

- Communities should be encouraged to govern and control their local health systems; healthcare providers should be accountable for the health status of their surrounding communities, not of individual patients.
- Plans to improve population health status will remain underfunded as long as they are driven by health marketplace interests.
- Most jobs available in economically disadvantaged neighborhoods are 20- or 30-hour-per-week jobs that do not provide health insurance. We must confront the public-policy underpinnings of employment issues affecting access to healthcare.

Economic Development and Job Creation

- Economically disadvantaged communities need jobs that offer stability; job retention and health-status improvement will follow.
- Economic-development money should be spent to help businesses with employment costs, because employers cannot keep up with the spiraling costs of insurance, taxes, and benefits.
- Many look to the health system as a source of jobs, because of the industry's size and because, in Chicago, many hospitals and health centers remain in communities that have been abandoned by other industries.

Housing

- When a two-flat is maintained in the neighborhood, the community is provided one unit of affordable home ownership along with one rental unit. Some public-housing problems can be avoided by landlords in two-flats: They can close their doors to tenants who undermine community stability.
- Pilot economic development strategies should be framed around the building of viable neighborhood real-estate markets. Real estate provides a good opportunity for a cottage industry based on local skill. Local residents can learn to maintain and enhance, and ultimately purchase two- and three-flat buildings on a modest income.
- Some tenant groups have invited people who have never entered public housing to visit informally with residents, increasing public appreciation of public-housing issues.

REFRAMED PERSPECTIVES ON COLLABORATION TO PROMOTE ECONOMIC DEVELOPMENT

Strategies for improving health in the community context are difficult to develop. Ultimately, they require organizational and governance structures as well as mechanisms for financing and mobilizing resources. They require leadership rising from the community. The following comments, again culled from the Sinai Health System town meeting, identify some current barriers to developing comprehensive community initiatives, as well as practices that could contribute to the success of future programs.

- Economic-development initiatives belong within a larger social-justice framework.
- When people feel abandoned, they become disillusioned and less able to handle or resolve conflicts. On an individual level, this can lead to problems with job retention. On a community level, it can block residents from coming together to develop solutions.
- Appropriate jurisdictions must be selected for planning large federally funded economic assistance initiatives. Regionalization should be key in planning local economic development and solving the problems of concentrated poverty in inner-city neighborhoods.
- Community development programs must be sustained long enough to allow new community leaders to be identified, nourished, and nurtured.
- Existing social programs and resources are invested in ways that do nothing to build the community as a healthy entity. Rather, social programs are designed to help isolated individuals. Each investment of this type pulls another thread from the fabric of the community, rather than tightening the weave.
- As communities develop, competing interests emerge, driving the community to expend energy on competition rather than on meeting the ultimate goal. A mechanism must be established to allow opposing power forces to resolve differences peaceably.
- One indicator of a healthy community is the degree to which the community is outspoken. Those with the greatest stake in their community naturally want to speak on their community's behalf.
- Money, leadership, and talent must recycle and remain in the community. This requires a commitment to stay and spend time in the community. Those who work but do not live in the community should be asked to reflect on the personal responsibility and leadership they could provide.
- As federal and state governments flounder in their efforts to set expenditure policies, money usually is invested in a variety of categorical programs. This does not accomplish as much as if the same resources were pooled and used to solve community problems.

THE GLASS HALF FULL

Kretzmann and McKnight (1993) and McKnight (1994) point out that most discussions on urban issues focus on the glass half empty rather than half full. Abundant studies describe what America's cities lack, but less clearly define the other half of the picture—what strategies are known to be effective.

Massive economic shifts during the past two decades have caused hundreds of thousands of industrial jobs to move away from the central city and its neighborhoods. Shifts in the economy and the disappearance of decent employment possibilities from low-income neighborhoods have removed the bottom rung from the fabled American ladder of opportunity. These circumstances require an unusual approach to critical urban questions such as how to assure decent housing and associated resource development.

Based on research in other cities, McKnight recommends that every institution in its neighborhood, whether a for-profit, not-for-profit, or government entity, should function as a "treasure chest" of resources for community building. Any sound development strategy should focus on how to open that treasure chest, understanding, for example, how parks, businesses, health systems, and the like can serve as a neighborhood resource. The ability to be a community resource requires knowledge of what works in the community.

Some town meeting voices reflecting on the glass half full included the following:

- Some urban conditions have changed, beginning about ten years ago and certainly swelling in the last five years. One is the economy based on drugs. The other is what neighborhood after neighborhood identifies as "a spiritual problem," or an issue of values, or a trust problem.

- One Chicago church created a rehabilitation effort for ex-offenders, drug offenders, and addicts, providing internship opportunities to men who had made commitments to turning their lives around, but who also needed work experience to build credibility as potential employees. Two factors contribute to this program's success. First, the interns were able to make use of the credibility they had within their church and could draw on moral support from the congregation. Second, they performed work the community needed.

- Some Chicago businesses maintain a "fort" mentality: They are in business despite the condition of the neighborhood. The city's industrial-corridor program has brought some people out of their forts and has encouraged responsibility and community outreach.

- Even tougher than funding issues are relationship issues. We must learn to ask about issues of race and the feelings that arise around this topic. If communities fail to address these issues, we will continue to die from within.

- One successful community housing development group had the foresight to appoint many of the community's dissenting voices to its board. This board has become the focal point for resolution of differences. As a result, development projects move forward.

The problems faced by disadvantaged communities are well known; needs surveys do not provide information adequate to the tasks faced by communities. The key question is not, "What are our needs and deficits," but rather, "What are we doing in our communities that helps us understand what will change it?" Health systems are among important stakeholders that are "doing something" in the community. In this sense, they are part of the treasure chest of resources that can be used to contribute to community development, economic improvement, and ultimately, improved community health status.

TOWARD THE ECONOMIC HEALTH OF COMMUNITIES

Within the last decade, both federal healthcare funding programs as well as private philanthropic grantmakers have tried to promote the building of partnerships and consortia as a means to improve community health and increase economic vitality. The Empowerment Zone program is emblematic of this trend, calling for collaborative neighborhood programs.

Through the Empowerment Zone process and other local collectives, healthcare providers have worked with neighboring local organizations to address public health and health access goals. Similarly, community development groups have joined together to define agendas for economic improvement. Given the inextricable linkage between health and economic security, health institutions such as Sinai Health System are wisely mobilizing to serve as partners in the development of local strategies to improve economic security, and in turn, to improve health.

Ultimately, however, the march of well-intentioned partners in search of solutions is destined to remain outside the mainstream of health care until we can better understand and address the effect of health within the economy in concrete terms. Within the healthcare provider community, no economic model exists to define how reinvestment of profit into community development creates a positive effect on the hospital's revenue base. Until hospitals can systematically relate community benefit to economic benefit within their institutions, and until they are driven by consumers to seek the logical basis for doing so, health systems that reach out to their communities as partners will lie outside of the mainstream, with no basis for translating into broader practice the type of creative, collaborative thinking typified by our town meeting participants.

For more information about Sinai Health System or the October 1995 forum, "Healing Bodies, Building Lives," contact the Public Affairs Office, Room N-325, California Avenue at 15th Street, Chicago, IL 60608, at (773) 257-6678.

REFERENCES

Greenspan, B. (1992). Mount Sinai: A special hospital for a special community. *Henry Ford Hosp Med J.*, *40*(1-2): 71–6.

Hojvat-Gallin, N. (1997). Ingredients of healthy communities. Working Paper. Health and Medicine Policy Research Group, Chicago.

Joseph, L. & Webber, H. (1995). *Medicaid in Illinois—Myths and realities.* Chicago: Metropolitan Planning Council and Health and Medicine Policy Research Group.

Kretzmann J. P. & McKnight, J. L. (1993). *Building communities from the inside out.* Chicago: ACTA Publications.

Manilow, S. (1994). Understanding what your community needs. *Trustee,* 47(3).

McKnight, J. (1994). Tools for well-being: Health systems and communities. *Am. J. Prev. Med.,* 100(suppl), 23–5.

Rodriguez-Trias, H. & Marte, C. (1994). Challenges and possibilities: Women, HIV and the healthcare system in the 1990s. In B. E. Schneider, N. E. Stoller (Eds.), *Women resisting AIDS: Feminist strategies of empowerment.* Philadelphia: Temple University Press.

Chapter 18

Transformational Leadership Development in Primary Health Care

SUSAN M. POSLUSNY

Promoting community transformation through leadership development is an important strategy in primary health care (PHC), and was the primary mission of the Leadership for Primary Health Care project (LPHC). Transformational leadership, as a concept, guided the design and implementation of the project. Transformational leadership development emerged as a model strategy that can contribute to health reform and social change. What is the nature of transformational leadership in disadvantaged communities and how does transformational leadership development contribute to social change and health reform? The main focus of this paper is a discussion of the conceptual ideas that emerged from the project. A brief discussion of the project is thus provided to ground the subsequent discussion of transformational leadership.

LEADERSHIP FOR
PRIMARY HEALTH CARE PROJECT

The LPHC project was funded for three years (1990–1993) by the W. K. Kellogg Foundation (see McElmurry et al., 1995). The project structure was developed to enhance the capacity for leadership in socioeconomically disadvantaged communities through collaborative partnerships between university personnel and community residents. The overall goal was to promote PHC as a strategy to achieve Health for All as defined by the Declaration of Alma Ata (World Health Organization, 1978).

Specifically, the project focused on the development of an action-learning program for grassroots community leaders and community-based health professionals. Project personnel included faculty and academic staff of the College of Nursing and the Department of Medical Education at the University of Illinois at Chicago (UIC). Program participants (fellows) representing the diverse ethnic communities of Chicago were nominated by grassroots community organizations or public sector institutions to attend a weekly workshop and develop a project focusing on PHC. Ultimately, forty-two fellows participated in the program representing twenty-six different community-based agencies.

The program included a curriculum for transformational leadership development in PHC, a teaching learning process designed to promote critical awareness, and support for community innovation and health policy development.

CURRICULUM FOR
TRANSFORMATIONAL LEADERSHIP

The leadership curriculum incorporated four assumptions about transformational education. First, there is strength in diversity. Fellows were chosen to participate in the program to represent the broad diversity in Chicago's ethnic communities and the multiple sectors involved in providing community-based health services. Second, learning occurs best through dialogue. All participants in the program were considered experts. Project personnel facilitated discussion within small groups. Group membership was purposely rearranged at intervals to encourage consideration of differing points of view. Third, there is empowerment with participation. Fellows were given the task of coming to consensus on selecting, designing, and implementing a group project that could benefit each of their communities. Although the negotiation process was long and arduous, the results of the group project gave most everyone a feeling of accomplishment and a desire to continue the project. Fourth, social change is the result of true partnerships. Partnerships extended beyond the classroom into the community as fellows developed individual projects to improve the health and well-being of their respective community areas with consultation from other fellows and project personnel.

TEACHING AND LEARNING FOR TRANSFORMATION

Empowerment education was selected as the teaching model for the program (Hope et al., 1984). Traditional education is built on a model of passive-receptive learning. Content is delivered through formal communication strategies. Students are expected to absorb the information without questioning its veracity or utility. With empowerment education, teaching is based on what learning needs are revealed through the process of developing critical awareness. For example, during a role play about communicating with a Korean grocer in an African-American community, learners are apt to reveal ethnic or racial stereotypes. Learners, or actors, then reflect on personal experiences for essential meanings and use the enhanced awareness to decide on future courses of action. Continuing with the previous example, learners may decide to explore reasons that Asian immigrants start businesses outside their own immigrant communities or why "Americans" resent foreign-born business owners. Often this exploration takes place within the diversity of the group; however, learners may decide to survey others or to go to a movie that depicts the particular situation. This translates into an educational process that encourages the student to pick the topics, design the strategies, and evaluate the outcomes of learning.

Workshops focused on building knowledge of successful leadership behaviors, primary health care strategies, community development, health resources management, information technology, and impact analysis. Skill-building exercises focused on team work, group negotiation, community assessment, program development, and participatory evaluation. The program fostered generic abilities in communication, social responsibility, cultural sensitivity, political savvy, planned change, and developing a vision. Project personnel and community fellows attended weekly workshops over the period of a year. Evaluation of the program was ongoing and predominantly qualitative in nature. Fellows described the substance and assessed the significance of their learning, and directed ongoing changes in the curriculum.

In the period since completing the leadership program, the author has reflected on some of the lessons learned about transformational leadership. In sharing these insights, it is important to first offer some background about transformational leadership before discussing our experiences within that context.

TRANSFORMATIONAL LEADERSHIP

Transformational leaders create and communicate a vision for change and empower others to take action and to become leaders themselves (Bennis & Nanus, 1985; Marriner-Tomey, 1993). A leader is defined as "one who has the ability to create a shared sense of reality and who plays a complementary role to the members in the leadership process" (Kosowski et al., 1990, p. 39). Leadership as an interactive process "enables all who participate to develop leadership skills in an atmosphere of shared power and mutual growth" (Kosowski et al., 1990, p. 36). Leaders *empower others* by their willingness to share in the processes of deciding, relating, influencing, and facilitating problem resolution. As a result, the entire group, as a distinct entity, is empowered as well.

Transformational leadership in the community is not always a matter of position, charisma, or legitimate authority (Roberts, 1985). Frequently, informal leadership emerges through various social relationships and organizations. These informal leaders are very recognizable to their peers as well as to the formal leadership in the community. They often live or work in the neighborhood and volunteer their time to help others. They are known by their abilities to recognize what needs to be done (critical awareness), demonstrate commitment, share decision making, organize others, build consensus, and work within existing systems to accomplish goals (practical action). These processes build upon each other to effect social change and health reform. (See Figure 1, Transformational Leadership Development.) Empowerment education, as a strategy to develop critical awareness, interacts with community partnerships to enhance transformational leadership abilities.

SPECIFIC ABILITIES OF TRANSFORMATIONAL LEADERS

1. **Promoting Critical Awareness.** Critical awareness is at the core of transformational leadership in communities. Critical awareness is a process whereby individuals reflect on personal experience and come to recognize the social reasons for their health problems and poor living conditions (Freire, 1968). Realizing that oppression is systematic and not random, and identifying the causes of oppression is empowering. Critical awareness evokes a strong emotional response to the identified injustices sufficient to provoke collective action. Vision of a better life emerges as people act to voice their needs and desires. Transformational leaders are skilled in helping people to gain critical awareness.

2. **Demonstrating Commitment.** The process of developing critical awareness helps build a commitment to benefit oneself and one's community (beneficence). In other words, commitment emerges as a consequence of significant life experience, personal relationships, and organizational affiliations that create critical awareness of the need for social change. In community organizations, commitment is demonstrated not simply in "doing your job" but in investing your energy to cause change (Bernstein, 1997).

Commitment goes beyond espousing popular values as in public politics. Commitment requires personal action in defense of those values. For example, there is a big difference between decrying the social waste of abandoned buildings (public politics) and spending a week renovating a building for low-income housing (commitment). Transformational leaders demonstrate strong personal commitment that can inspire others to effect social change (Roberts, 1985).

Personal commitment can empower individuals and groups to tackle difficult social agendas. However, strong personal commitments also can create boundaries of exclusion across individuals and groups, frequently referred to as "turf," that can splinter community efforts. Transformational leaders recognize the multiple commitments that diverse groups bring to the negotiating table or the classroom and can build consensus despite differing agendas.

3. **Negotiating a Uniform Group Response**. Building consensus means being able to support and enact group decisions. It does not necessarily require reaching total agreement. Finding common goals and shared values is essential in building consensus. Making decisions using an appropriate process is also essential in consensus building. Choice of decision making process should be made based on the degree of conflict and personal involvement in the situation. The transformational leader can assess the situation, help individual members articulate their goals and values, and negotiate a process for decision making. Through this process, the transformational leader encourages commitment to a group agenda.

4. **Making Shared Decisions**. Shared decision making is a powerful tool that invests people in the outcome of their decisions. Participation in PHC goes beyond simple investment of time and energy to accomplish tasks. Community participation means involving residents in deciding what should be done, how to do it, and who should be responsible. Transformational leaders enable others to make decisions and to act on those decisions. Most important, transformational leaders accept the outcomes of the shared decision-making process.

5. **Energizing Others**. Organizing others into action depends on a clear goal and the ability to reach that goal. Knowing what needs to change and having a visionary goal are not sufficient to organize groups into action. An effective community organizer can define a specific objective that can be accomplished within a reasonable amount of time. In addition, the objective should be attainable with available means. "If we only had money," is the most common complaint and reason for inaction. Strategies need to be relatively simple, uniform, and focused. It should be very easy to explain why and how someone should get involved. It also should be very easy to know when you have accomplished your goal. The transformational leader communicates the objective publicly and consistently, and inspires others by example to work tirelessly in its accomplishment.

6. **Transforming Ideas into Action**. Transformational leaders can transform ideas into action. Practical, theory-driven action (or praxis) is the point at which theory and practice meet to effect social change. Praxis is reached when the force of conviction becomes so powerful that people are driven to act in the defense of their beliefs. Revolution is the classic example of praxis. More typical examples perhaps are voting, letter writing, and volunteering. Praxis is the logical outcome of critical awareness.

COMMUNITY INNOVATION

There are a number of legitimate reasons why it is more difficult to implement transformational leadership in disadvantaged communities. Often, such communities have been the focus of improvement projects designed by academics and professionals who do not normally live in or interact with the community. When their externally driven projects result in no real or lasting change for community residents, a cycle of raised hopes, disappointment, and lasting mistrust is repeated. Each time a community is disappointed, trust diminishes and it is harder to elicit participation and hope in the ultimate benefit of a new project. Community organizations that operate on a shoestring budget often lack the resources to secure funding from major foundations or government groups. Using "simpler technologies" is not a matter of choice but a lack of funds to access and maintain more complex technologies. Lack of meaningful information, adequate education, and a viable job economy serves to further disempower community members. Inadequate community resources such as transportation, police protection, and public parks enforce isolation. Diminished opportunities to interact with a variety of individuals from different social groups and/or more economically privileged communities ultimately restricts the community resident's vision of a better future.

Poslusny et al. (1992) reported a number of shortcomings in classical diffusion theory especially when it was applied to "traditional" versus "modern" social structures. According to Rogers, diffusion of innovation is more difficult in traditional social systems (e.g., disadvantaged communities) than in modern social systems (e.g., prosperous communities). Traditional social systems are characterized by (1) adherence to maintaining the status quo and resistance to change, (2) use of "simpler technologies," (3) low levels of literacy and formal education, (4) heavy emphasis on the maintenance of family and other personal relationships, (5) little communication outside the social system, and (6) difficulty envisioning new roles or nontraditional social relationships (1971). Rogers makes no effort to explain these characteristics from the perspective of the community itself.

Developing critical awareness of the real causes of this separation between traditional and modern social systems helps to guide community transformation projects. Rogers (1973) wrote that while successful innovation is largely determined by "top-down" leadership, "power elites act as gatekeepers to prevent restructuring innovations from entering a social system, while favoring functioning innovations that do not immediately threaten to change the system's structure" (p. 76). In reality, stable bureaucracies, such as the traditional health-care system, are less susceptible to grassroots efforts for health reform and will only support change that benefits the continued existence of the organization. The greatest threat to community innovation is from the power elites outside local neighborhoods who refuse to relinquish control of funding decisions and program plans to community organizations. There is greater likelihood of successful innovation when existing organizations and their constituencies can share control and derive equal benefit from its adoption (i.e., partnerships between professionals, community residents, and community leaders can facilitate community transformation and improve health systems). As awareness of the disparity in access to healthcare grows, there is more support for innovation in healthcare delivery at the local level. Local action is more successful in traditional communities than imposed change. Therefore, health system changes and innovation at the community level is more likely to be accomplished by grassroots efforts.

Communities involved in the LPHC project were characterized as traditional social systems or disadvantaged communities. The educational program, in focusing on building resources and personal capacity for leadership, encouraged the development of grassroots innovation in a number of areas. Successful fellows' projects emphasized environmental justice, economic development, jobs creation, youth empowerment, and women as the primary source of healing in the community. Affiliated relationships in the family and neighborhood both represented the status quo and were viewed as purveyors of harmony and balance in the community. Leadership trainees provided materials to enhance informational resources. Access to current technology and information was improved by developing a clearinghouse for materials about PHC and community development. Work space with a personal computer helped introduce fellows to word processing and desktop publishing. Fellows enjoyed field trips to organizations outside their community area, such as the city planning department and donors forum. The role of project personnel was to engage and support community relationships in the process of developing PHC outcomes that were affordable, culturally acceptable, practical, scientifically sound, and universally accessible.

HEALTH POLICY DEVELOPMENT

Insuring that communities would benefit from leadership activities was a guiding principle in the administration of the project; however, sustaining the benefits of community-based projects is often difficult. Professionally driven models of healthcare innovation have personnel costs that are a strain on the limited budgets of most community organizations. Further, equity issues are raised if projects expect participation of volunteers from the community while health professionals expect salaries.

The LPHC project budget was designed to ensure financial as well as professional resources for the organizations and individuals who participated. As a result, resources were available to a number of community areas in Chicago that had a demonstrated need for leadership, education, innovation, and health innovation. Fellows received stipends for their participation in workshops. Nominating organizations received funds to support the projects that fellows developed. Project resources were used to fund the group project. In addition, by focusing on building talent and capacity for leadership within the community, many participants were able to sustain the projects they had developed and the majority of fellows remained in their communities.

OUTCOMES OF TRANSFORMATIONAL LEADERSHIP DEVELOPMENT

In the current climate of cost containment in healthcare, there are critical questions that need to be asked about the project in assessing its impact on the community as a whole. What contribution to health reform was made? Is transformational leadership better than other styles of leadership? Did the health status of the communities improve as the result of the project? Do partnerships help traditional social structures benefit from innovation? The answers are not definitive.

HEALTHCARE REFORM

Health care is an evolving phenomenon. In the early 1990s, hopes for a national healthcare plan were high. A Health Security Act had been proposed that emphasized PHC. There was even anticipation that funding would be available for community initiatives like those developed in the project. Since that time however, healthcare reform initiatives have been sidelined and for-profit organizations have taken over the healthcare system. This takeover includes obscene salaries to CEOs and shareholders who insist on profitable bottom lines for the parent corporations employing healthcare providers. Managed care membership is mandated for a growing majority of Medicare and Medicaid recipients. It is questionable whether managed care organizations will accept their responsibility to return some of their profits from Medicare and Medicaid tax dollars to the communities (Showstack et al., 1996).

The public sector has the primary responsibility to provide resources at the grassroots level to promote PHC and achieve Health for All. However, multisectoral collaboration (i.e., give-and-take among individuals across geographic and institutional boundaries) is an equally important dimension of PHC. Transformational leadership development is one approach that can inform efforts of public health and managed care organizations to improve the health of communities.

ETHICAL LEADERSHIP

The best practices of leadership are elusive. In order to determine best practices, one has to identify the desired outcome. Is the outcome financial gain, community benefits, or resource equity? Is the need so critical as to require expediency in achieving the desired outcomes? There are a variety of leadership styles. Autocratic leadership exerts a great deal of control over the goals and actions of their constituencies. Critical need or economic motivation frequently demands a very results-oriented leader. Over time however, the constituency will become increasingly passive and resentful of autocratic leaders. Charismatic leaders motivate and influence others to *want* to follow. Charismatic leaders are capable of positive or negative influence. The ability to sustain outcomes over time, when community activities are tied to the qualities of the charismatic leader, can be jeopardized when the leader leaves or is deposed. Democratic leadership can be very expedient and provide for the continuing survival of the group, not just the leader. Democracy is based on the assumption of equality and independence of all members in the constituency, which is an assumption that is only partly true in society.

Current literature emphasizes vision and the ethical dimension of leadership (i.e., effective leaders share their power with their constituents). Kouzes and Posner (1995) describe this as "encouraging the heart." The best practices of transformational leaders draw on the values, aspirations, and skills of all members in the leadership process to achieve mutually desired goals. Process is emphasized. Outcomes are achieved, but not necessarily by the most direct route. While transformational leadership may not be expedient, it is a means to achieve equitable and improved social status for members in the leadership process.

COMMUNITY HEALTH IMPROVEMENT

The health status of a community, as an outcome of transformational leadership, is extremely difficult to measure. There are numerous tools and clinical protocols that can be used to assess the health status of individuals. These measurements can be very sensitive to subtle changes in the health of individuals. However, indicators of community health status are much less sensitive. The health of incredibly large numbers of individuals must be affected in order to make a significant difference in commonly used community health status indicators (e.g., accidental death rate). Excess and unnecessary deaths will not succumb to a "germ theory" model of prevention. There is no pill for preventing excess deaths.

It is doubtful that any one project will cause measurable change in community health status indicators. However, if a handful of adolescents are prevented from joining gangs because of a community outreach center program, the impact can be enormous for a community. Other children will not be killed in gang violence. These children will have the opportunity to get an education, become productive members of society, and serve as role models to future generations. The accidental death rate will not change by very much. The infant mortality rate will not register a change. People will still die. The overall impact on community health will be diffuse rather than concentrated on one indicator of health status which has even greater potential for fundamental social change.

SOCIAL CHANGE

Communities in urban America are in constant transition. Increased mobility, gentrification, declining birth rates, new immigrants, loss of federal entitlements, and erosion of the job market are examples of factors that are forcing communities in contemporary society to find new ways to balance its resources and needs.

Failure or inability to innovate in response to these demands places communities, and the people who live in them, in crisis on a daily basis. Violence, drug use, unemployment, and child neglect are the well-publicized signs of that daily crisis.

The traditional approach in healthcare and community development has been to focus on the most glaring needs or deficits of the individuals in a community and to provide problem-specific services. Higher rates of low birth weight are met with additional prenatal care programs. Teen pregnancy is answered with sex education and free condoms. Child abuse is countered with parenting classes.

Just as repeated abortions are a poor solution to the need for family planning, resolving urgent community problems only on a case-by-case (or problem-by-problem) basis is ultimately inadequate because the resource base is never sufficiently developed to prevent recurrence of the problems. As a result, problems such as substance abuse, teen pregnancy, premature death, and disability continue to be endemic in the urban community.

Partnerships between community residents and health professionals are thought to improve access to PHC, thereby creating the potential for social

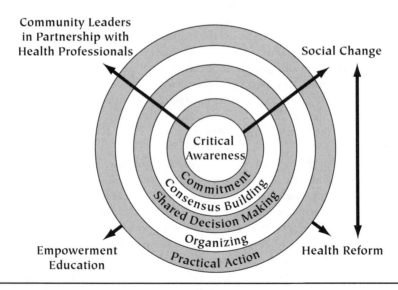

FIGURE 1.
Transformational Leadership Development

change (Bless et al., 1995; Courtney et al., 1996; Lenihan, 1993). However, partnerships alone are not enough. Programs in primary prevention and specific protection against disease, while essential, are not sufficient to alter the socioeconomic factors that maintain poor health outcomes in many of our nation's communities. Leadership is needed to access the individual talents and organizational commitments that can drive and sustain community transformation. Effective partnerships in traditional communities are dependent on the abilities and commitment of individuals and groups to work together. The ability of individuals to transform themselves from the separate roles of leader and follower to complementary roles is essential. In order to work together, organizations must restrict their ambitions for recognition as the singular expert or gatekeeper and develop missions that are more consultative and collaborative. In essence, a partnership relationship should eliminate the need to exercise power in defense of personal or organizational turf. As such, there is a great deal more hope in breaking down barriers to innovation in traditional communities when goals are approached by partners rather than competitors and when critical awareness informs the partnership.

REFLECTIONS

Upon reflection, the LPHC project was able to promote community transformation because it took a comprehensive, community development approach to PHC and health reform, not because it targeted specific diseases or deficits in the community. Emphasis was on broad social change as well as individual benefit. Health was defined broadly to include social and economic dimensions in addition to biomedical dimensions. Participation in the project was broad with representation from a number of community areas in the city. Leadership development strategies emphasized process and principles of collaboration, mutual benefits, and shared resources. Teaching and learning strategies emphasized critical awareness, shared decision making, consensus building, and practical action. Innovation was encouraged through partnerships rather than technical assistance. Most important for grassroots health policy development, the project emphasized the development of vision for a better future.

REFERENCES

Bennis, W. & Nanus, B. (1985). *Leaders: The strategies for taking charge.* New York: Harper & Row.

Bernstein, P. (1997). *Best practices of effective non-profit organizations.* New York: The Foundation Center.

Bless, C., Murphy, D., & Vinson, N. (1995). Nurses' role in primary health care. *Nursing & Health Care: Perspectives on Community, 16*(2), 70–76.

Courtney, R., Ballard, E., Fauver, S., Gariota, M. & Holland, L. (1996). The partnership model: Working with individuals, families, and communities toward a new vision of health. *Public Health Nursing, 13*(3), 177–186.

Freire, P. (1968). *Pedagogy of the oppressed*. New York: Seabury Press.

Hope, A. & Timmel, S. (1984). *Training for transformation: A handbook for community workers*. Gweru, Zimbabwe: Mambo Press.

Kouzes, J. & Posner, B. (1995). *The leadership challenge: How to keep getting things done in organizations* (2nd ed.). San Francisco: Jossey-Bass.

Kosowski, M., Grabbe, L., Grams, K., Lobb, M., Willoughby, D., Davis, S., & Simes, G.(1990). An interactive model of leadership. *Nursing Administration Quarterly, 15*(1), 36–43.

Lenihan, P., Ferguson, R., & Terrell, P. (1993). Health care reform in Chicago: Melding global thought with local action. *Journal of Ambulatory Care Management, 16*(4), 60–66.

McElmurry, B. J., Tyska, C., Gugenheim, A. M., Misner, S., & Poslusny, S. (1995). Leadership for primary health care. *Nursing & Health Care: Perspectives on Community, 16*(4), 229-33.

Marriner-Tomey, A. (1993). *Transformational leadership development in nursing*. St. Louis: Mosby.

Poslusny, S., Swider, S., Newcomb, J., & McElmurry, B. J. (1992, August 6). *Information diffusion and utilization of women's health research in primary health care*. Paper presented at the International State of the Science Congress, Washington, D.C.

Roberts, N. (1985). Transforming leadership: A process of collective action. *Human Relations, 38*(11), 1023–1046.

Rogers, E. M. (1973). Social structure and social change. In G. Zaltman (Ed.), *Processes and phenomena of social change*. New York: Wiley & Sons.

Rogers, E. M. (1983). *Diffusion of innovations* (3rd ed.). New York: Free Press.

Rogers, E. M. & Shoemaker, F. F. (1971). *Communication of innovations* (2nd ed.). New York: Free Press.

Showstack, J., Lurie, N. Leatherman, S. Fisher, E., & Inui, T. (1996). Health of the public: The private-sector challenge. *Journal of the American Medical Association, 276*(13), 1071–1074.

World Health Organization (1978). *Primary health care: A joint report by the Director-General of the World Health Organization and the Executive Director of the United Nations Children's Fund*. Geneva: World Health Organization.

Chapter 19

Lessons Learned

BEVERLY J. MCELMURRY
with the assistance of
RANDY SPREEN PARKER
CYNTHIA TYSKA
TODD HISSONG

Throughout this book, authors of the various chapters have shared what they learned in the process of planning, implementing, and evaluating their program and/or project. For us to arrive at an overall summary of the lessons learned from various projects, two meetings were convened to discuss the ideas that selected authors wanted to share with readers. The group invited to meet with us were the professionals (primarily women) who had held major leadership positions in various primary health care (PHC) projects or programs (Peg Dublin, Ada Mary Gugenheim, Agatha Lowe, Beverly J. McElmurry, Susan Misner, Joan Newcomb, Kathleen Norr, Chang Gi Park, Randy Spreen Parker, Susan Poslusny, Sue Swider, and Cynthia Tyska). Each meeting lasted three to four hours and was recorded and transcribed. These lively conversations were shared with the group participants for further feedback. Subsequently, the authors of this chapter identified a list of the lessons learned and grouped them in six major themes: *Effectiveness, participatory process, community expertise, continuing education, collaborative decisions,* and *sustainability.* Like all things characteristic of this effort to capture PHC in action, the following categorizations should be viewed as a working document.

LESSONS LEARNED

I. PHC is an effective strategy for health reform in urban communities.

  A. Urban community health development occurs in a constantly changing political, economic, and social environment.
  B. The provision of essential health services is basic to urban development.
  C. Societal shifts in thinking about PHC take time.

Discussion

We asked the discussion group to make global conclusions that reflected their insights based on several years of work in the field. The group was encouraged to remain true to our conceptualization of PHC attributes while recognizing that in reality there are constant negotiations and concessions between desired and realized goals. In developing this book, we had urged each author to include in their respective chapters the lessons they had learned from their projects. Therefore, while we do make some general comments here that may refer to a given chapter, we do so for illustrative purposes rather than pointing out all of the lessons the individual authors indentified. Most authors of the chapters presented earlier in this book attest to the effectiveness of their PHC efforts. However, Barton's description of an urban teaching clinic (Chapter 11) illustrates that one can effectively integrate PHC into a health provider–driven setting, and supports our conviction that individual healthcare providers can make a difference when their overall PHC philosophy coalesces with their daily primary care practice.

Although primary care practitioners are usually working with small numbers of individuals or families, their work is significant when it fuels the larger community organizational efforts and grounds the professionals in the reality of their clients. Further, such individuals can convey the philosophy of PHC to health professions students who train at urban community-based health centers. To achieve this reorientation of health professions students to PHC, it is important that students experience firsthand the realities of the community's residents as well as the realities of a health center that respects its constituents and their needs.

II. Effective PHC requires the implementation of a participatory process for shared decision making.

    A. Collaboration requires shared authority and power relationships between community members and health professionals.

    B. Partnerships between university and community-based settings challenge the traditions of the university by emphasizing that community residents share in the decision-making activities that affect them.

    C. Community-based PHC initiatives necessitate a change in attitudes, styles, and the personal growth of health professionals.

    D. In establishing agendas for health, community residents must participate fully in the design, implementation, and evaluation of their health and health care.

Discussion

Critical consciousness (as explored by many of the previous chapter authors) is an effective teaching and learning strategy for transformational leadership development with residents of low-income, underserved urban communities. Involving both community leaders and health professionals from a variety of different ethnic communities in program activities enhances the learning of all participants.

Many authors in the preceding chapters express concern that the outcomes of programs—whether it be their impact on the community, contribution to improved community health status, or effect on community leadership—are often known only after a lengthy period of time. Further, those programs that do actually obtain funding for evaluation studies are often hampered by requirements to focus on immediate impacts (i.e., ideational or action-based descriptions) that do not capture longitudinal changes. Several chapters deal with these evaluation issues, some challenge our traditional analyses (Soares et al., Chapter 3; Norr et al., Chapter 6) and others illustrate that follow-up assessments do support the observation that projects have longitudinal and lasting changes.

Engaging a select group of community residents to critically question, analyze, and act upon their situation requires a certain focus. For example, when university personnel are engaged in training community members, it is imperative to keep an open dialogue with them and constantly try to understand and appreciate their real-life experiences. When these efforts are combined with educational activities that truly engage both instructor and student, community residents begin to engage in critical thinking. While critical thinking is most successful when community members are discussing their own experiences, planned activities are needed as well to generalize critical thinking situations that are relevant, yet unfamiliar, to their lives. Having students of different ethnicity in the same class and engaging them through their culture greatly enriches the learning experience of all students.

III. **Urban community residents seek participation in PHC that is consistent with their characteristics/skills.**

   A. Community residents seek strategies to develop their abilities to respond to the health needs of their community and have their voices heard by health professionals and policy makers.
   B. PHC is valued by community residents because this strategy recognizes that health is interrelated with all aspects of life.

Discussion

While we indicated that communities seek participation in PHC activities, Reed (Chapter 10) illustrates that introducing any new idea or behavior into a community will not necessarily be welcomed or integrated immediately because individuals, groups, and the community as a whole have their established modes of practice. It takes a great deal of time, effort, and acceptance of people's established ways to achieve assimilation of new ideas or behaviors into established practices. Even though capacity-building concepts and asset development tools are common in many projects, these concepts challenge the cultural norms of communities and the everyday practices of their residents. The power of participation in PHC is highlighted in the advocates report of their development over time (Norr et al., Chapter 4), and by the empowerment and social value described by the recipients of these services (Buck and Fox, Chapter 5; Park and Warren, Chapter 7).

IV. **PHC requires the ongoing development and education of stakeholders.**

   A. It takes time to develop trusting and productive relationships between university/community collaborators in health activities.
   B. Effective community participation in PHC requires that stakeholders develop knowledge about health, consumer rights, resource procurement and management, program planning and evaluation, and community development and mobilization.
   C. Valid and reliable community-based health research/evaluation requires that community residents understand the importance of participating in research design, development, and implementation.
   D. Preparing community residents for participation in PHC activities is an ongoing and personnel-intensive process.

Discussion

It is important for a university to enhance community health and development in low-income, underserved areas by helping to develop its leaders and potential innovators. Long after their engagement with a university-based educational program, these leaders remain in their community. Chapter 18 (Poslusny) focuses on transformational leadership and a specific educational program to develop individual and community capacities, as well as address individual, community, and social issues. An individual leader's personal needs (and those of their communities) are best served through a program that focuses on innovation, decision making and practical action. Partnership, collaboration, mutual benefits, shared resources, and consensus-building are the tools that create harmony and effective teamwork.

Shapiro and Greenspan (Chapter 17) describe several examples of how traditional hospital/health institutions can redefine their institutional perspective on providing care using a definition of health that incorporates economic development and job creation as well as housing. The subsequent establishment of a network of community-based clinics can help hospitals to maintain an essential connection to local communities and neighborhoods.

V. **Effective PHC initiatives realize consensus on the criteria that participants use for judging quality outcomes.**

   A. The focus of PHC programs addresses the health issues and interests of community residents.
   B. The realization of healthier communities represents a focus on improving health indicators and building community capacity for dealing with health-relevant areas.
   C. PHC programs require a broad and diverse range of participants and skills.

Discussion

A broad perspective on health, one that includes social and economic dimensions in addition to biomedical areas, encompasses the real issues of different communities involved in PHC. Interestingly, community residents often grasp the importance of viewing wellness within a broad health and development framework more quickly than their professional counterparts. Many authors addressed the importance of recognizing the culture and language of the participants as well as their geographic identification when launching health programs. These are central factors in determining how to engage them in personal decision making about health and community capacity building (Ramos and Ramos, Chapter 12). Multidisciplinary groups bring different professional cultures to a setting. This is particularly clear in school-based programs where educators, health professionals, and community residents must learn to blend their differing perspectives and priorities.

VI. Sustaining PHC initiatives is an ongoing challenge.

A. Health advocacy efforts with families, individuals, and communities require comprehensive and multifocused programs.

B. A focus on PHC is contrary to the tendency of our government to fund categorical and problem-oriented health initiatives.

C. Sustaining a PHC delivery system will require creative use of existing funds and fundamental changes in the allocation of existing funds for health services.

Discussion

Leadership development and sustainability are essential to the success of PHC initiatives. Both community residents and health professionals need more formally structured ways to identify, nurture, and support the talents of potential leaders, particularly in the development of community capacity and organizational support for community leaders. Individuals develop leadership skills through the groups or efforts they join, and this experiential component is critical to theorizing about or testing community-based activities.

It remains a challenge to find the best means to measure the synergistic effect of collaborative activities and the value that all stakeholders ascribe to a PHC service. Thus, even when one achieves some success in combining outcome measures with process components embedded in the context of participants, sometimes even the most successful programs may not be sustainable. How to convince policy makers to invest in PHC strategies is as challenging as convincing funders that some processes take time to evolve naturally and do not fit the traditional structure/mold of predetermined outcomes.

In closing, we learned from all contributing authors (and through our own experiences) a basic, undeniable lesson: Creating productive teams with the necessary skills, knowledge, and values to implement PHC requires the patience of a saint, supportive environments, understanding funders, and a measure of good luck. Fortunately, we have been lucky to find participants who share our commitment to changing health care. In particular, changes that ensure essential health care for all that is equitable, accessible, acceptable, resource friendly, culturally sensitive, and attentive to participation by individuals, intersectoral cooperation, and continuity of care. Working within an urban PHC framework continues to be a challenging and rewarding experience.

Index